Brahmi

(*Bacopa monniera*)

Activities and Applications of the Versatile Ayurvedic Herb

Saligrama C. Subbarao

Lakshmi Subbarao

Bruce Ferguson

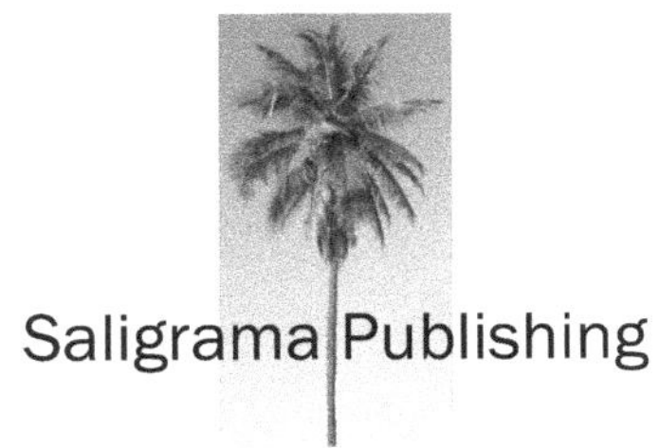

Published by Saligrama Publishing.

Contact the primary author at saligrama_subbarao@yahoo.com

ISBN 978-0-9843812-2-7

Printed in the United States of America

I warmly dedicate this book to

My friend Dr. Leland Dale Smucker (1935-2011), a large hearted and broad minded person

and

My nephew Jagannath Govindaraju (1958-2013), an avid reader, selfless helper of the needy, and modest person

-SCS

Acknowledgments

From *Saligrama Subbarao:*

First and foremost, I want to thank all of the scientists for their dedication to Brahmi research and published work. Without their contributions, this book could not have been written.

My coauthors Lakshmi Subbarao and Bruce Ferguson deserve special thanks. Lakshmi drew on her extensive analytical chemistry experience to revise multiple drafts of the manuscript, improving its content and format. She completed the arduous task of generating the structures in Chapter 2. She examined the numerous references and organized them into a manageable form. Her exceptional skills as a project manager kept everyone on the same page, and her passion and dedication to her work motivated the coauthors to do their part. Bruce reviewed each chapter carefully and made a number of appropriate additions and deletions. His rich and varied experience in the nutraceutical industry was invaluable to the preparation of this book.

I would like to thank my family for their genuine interest and invaluable assistance. My wife Mythili provided both unconditional support to complete the task, as well as frequent reminders to do so in a timely manner. Along with the other roles played by my children Kartik and Lakshmi in the writing of this book, their overwhelming encouragement was continually energizing. I want to thank my sisters, Vedavathi Govindaraju, Manjula Laxminarasimhiah and Shambhavi Vijayasarathy, my late brother Athri Sharma's wife Jayashree, and my niece Deepika Sharma for their superb hospitality while I was researching this book in Bengaluru.

I want to thank my friend Prof. Mahinder Chopra and his wife Swaran Chopra for their encouragement. I would also like to thank Mr. R. Shivashankar for his interest in this work and encouragement. Special thanks to Dr. Robert Abel, whose holistic attitude to the treatment of patients is an inspiration.

I would like to thank Dr. Dinesh Agrawal, Professor, Penn State University, for his help. I wish to express my gratitude to Dr. S. B. Krupanidhi, Professor, Indian Institute of Science, Bengaluru, and Dr. B. R. Ramakrishna, Principal, Sushruta Ayurveda Medical College, Bengaluru, for permitting me to use their libraries.

I am especially thankful to my friend Dr. K. Ramachandra Bhat for reading the book draft and offering helpful advice, suggestions and constructive comments. My sincere thanks to my friend Dr. Amar Tung for reading the book draft and making helpful suggestions. I would like to thank Dr. Daniel Lee for helping to obtain a number of articles and discussing various aspects of neurodegenerative disorders. I would like to thank Dr. Robert Langley for his encouragement.

I would like to thank my nephews Jagannath Govindaraju and Meghanath Laxminarasimhiah for their invaluable contributions. Jagannath took me to various places in India where Brahmi is grown, and helped me obtain a large number of reference materials from libraries. His untimely death in 2013 was a severe shock to me, and stilled my work for some time. As I reflected on his service to society and the unstinted support that he gave me personally, my vigor to complete the book was renewed. Meghanath accompanied me to several libraries while I was in Bengaluru. He typed a few chapters of this book and carefully supervised the typing of other chapters.

Finally, I would like to thank Kartik Subbarao, Chief Editor of Saligrama Publishing. He played a pivotal role in this endeavor. His patient and tireless efforts made the publication of this book possible. He meticulously read numerous drafts of the manuscript and thoroughly edited them. He also designed the organization and layout of the book.

Preface

Plants have been used for medicinal purposes since ancient times. In Ayurveda, the traditional system of Indian medicine, medicinal plants and herbs play a central role. It is estimated that 70-95% of the population in developing countries relies on traditional medicines, of which herbal products are essential components[1]. In recent years, the use of herbal products has increased enormously in the US, Europe, Australia and other regions throughout the world. In the US, about 17.7% of adults used herbal products in 2007[2], and sales of herbal supplements reached nearly $5.6 billion in 2012[3]. Globally, the herbal supplement market is projected to reach $107 billion by 2017[4]. A number of factors have helped to boost consumer confidence in herbal supplements, including the availability of high quality products.

Over the last few decades, a considerable amount of work has been done to scientifically validate the efficacy of a number of herbs. One herb that has received a lot of attention is Brahmi (Bacopa monniera). Extensive in vitro, in vivo and clinical studies on various effects of Brahmi have been conducted, and the results have been published in a wide variety of professional journals and other media worldwide. This book provides in one place the results of a number of significant investigations. Its intent is to serve as an accessible reference and guide for formulators, R&D professionals, biomedical researchers and medical practitioners.

The book is divided into 21 chapters. The first chapter provides a brief introduction to Ayurveda and the cultivation of Brahmi. The second chapter deals with its constituents and analysis. Chapters 3 to 20 address the various effects. Chapter 21 summarizes safety-related issues and provides concluding remarks.

I became interested in this topic after I retired from academia at the age of 69. I began pondering over the numerous health issues that people face as they age. Although many of them can be prevented or remedied, some of them are intractable. For example, Alzheimer's disease (AD) is a currently incurable disease that has confounded researchers.

Witnessing friends succumb to AD motivated me to diligently research the disease in both conventional and Ayurvedic medical literature. I learned that Ayurveda has plenty to offer in the treatment of AD, such as herbs that have the potential to reverse behavioral deficits and pathology. Brahmi is one of those magnificent herbs. It not only acts as an excellent nootropic agent, but also exerts, as I would discover, a number of other therapeutic effects.

The idea of writing a book on this marvelous plant dawned on me. I sought the help of my daughter Lakshmi Subbarao, a talented analytical chemist, and Bruce Ferguson, a long-time friend with a background in alternative medicine and over 25 years of experience in the nutraceutical industry. They worked alongside me with great enthusiasm and commitment to complete this work.

References

1 Molly Meri Robinson and Xiaorui Zhang. The World Medicines Situation 2011, Traditional Medicines: Global Situation, Issues and Challenges. World Health Organization, Geneva, 2011.

2 Patricia M Barnes, Barbara Bloom, Richard L Nahin. "CDC National Health Statistics Report #12. Complementary and Alternative Medicine Use Among Adults and Children: United States, 2007". National Institutes of Health, 2008.

3 American Botanical Council. Herbal Dietary Supplement Retail Sales Up 5.5% in 2012. http://cms.herbalgram.org/press/2013/2012_Market_Report.html

4 Global Herbal Supplements and Remedies Market to Reach US $107 Billion by 2017, According to New Report by Global Industry Analysts, Inc., 2012. http://prweb.com/releases/herbal_supplements/herbal_remedies/prweb9260421.htm

Table of Contents

1 - Introduction....1
2 - Constituents and Analysis....15
3 - Antioxidant Activity....39
4 - Nootropic Activity....65
5 - Antiamnesic Activity....85
6 - Effect on Alzheimer's Disease (AD)....91
7 - Effect on Parkinson's Disease (PD)....103
8 - Anxiolytic and Antidepressant Activity....113
9 - Effect on ADHD and ASD....123
10 - Anticonvulsant Activity....131
11 - Immunomodulatory Activity....141
12 - Anti-inflammatory Activity....149
13 - Antistress Activity....157
14 - Antidiabetic Activity....163
15 - Antiulcer Activity....167
16 - Liver and Kidney Protective Activity....175
17 - Cardioprotective Activity....183
18 - Effect on Cancer....187
19 - Antimicrobial Activity....197
20 - Other Effects....205
21 - Safety-Related Issues and Conclusion....215
Common Abbreviations....221

1 – Introduction

1.1 – General

Brahmi is a renowned medicinal plant. It is a household name in India, where its use for improving concentration, learning and memory goes back several thousand years. This plant has many names in Sanskrit, but the name Brahmi holds special significance. In Hindu mythology, Brahma is the creator of the universe, and his consort Brahmi (well known as Saraswati) is the goddess of learning. Perhaps this amazing plant was called Brahmi because of its capacity for improving cognitive functions[1]. Brahmi is mentioned in Vedic scriptures as old as 5000 BC[2]. In the gurukuls (residential schools or Ashrams) of ancient India, students were given Brahmi to enhance their ability to remember lengthy Vedic hymns and epics which were orally transmitted[3]. To this day, newborns are anointed with Brahmi with the hope of improving their intelligence, to open the "gates of Brahma"[4]. Brahmi's other Sanskrit names include Nirbrahmi, Brahmacarini, Jalanimba, Jalabrahmi, Divya, Saraswati, Aindri, Medhya, Bharati, Soma, Sharada, Surashrestha, Brahmakamya and Kapotavanka[5] (names in other Indian languages are presented in section 1.5). Brahmi's English names include Herb of grace, Water hyssop, and Thyme-leafed gratiola. The botanical name for Brahmi is *Bacopa monniera* (or *monnieri*) (L.) Pennell.

The therapeutic benefits of Brahmi have been well established in Ayurveda, the traditional system of Indian medicine. The next few sections present background information on Ayurveda, to provide context for the various applications of Brahmi.

1.2 – Overview of Ayurveda

Ayurveda, which means "science of life" in Sanskrit, is a comprehensive health care system that originated in India more than 5000 years ago[6]. It is a holistic approach designed to help people attain a state of physical, mental, social and spiritual well being. Ayurveda's philosophy is to treat the whole person, not just superficial symptoms. The primary focus is on preventing disease while preserving and promoting health[7]. It also offers a variety of therapies to treat illness.

Ayurveda is based on the panchamahabhuta (five great elements) theory. According to this theory, the entire universe - including human beings, animals, plants and lifeless things - is composed of five "Mahabhutas" symbolically represented by Akasha (space), Vayu (air), Apo (water), Teja (Fire) and Prithvi (earth).

1.2.1 - Doshas

The mahabhutas interact with each other and manifest in the body as Tridoshas (three types of life forces): Vata, Pitta and Kapha. Each dosha is a combination of two of the five mahabhutas and is associated with specific body functions as summarized below (Table 1.1):

Dosha	Components	Associated Function
Vata	Akasha (space) and Vayu (air)	All voluntary and involuntary movements in the body such as respiration, blood circulation, heartbeat, nerve conduction, blinking of the eye, etc.
Pitta	Teja (fire) and Apo (water)	Digestive and metabolic activities, regulation of body temperature, complexion, visual perception, hunger and thirst.
Kapha	Apo (water) and Prithvi (earth)	Provides strength and stability for holding tissues together; lubricates, moistens and maintains immunity.

Table 1.1: Doshas and their associated functions

Each person has all three doshas in a specific ratio. The proportion in which the three doshas are expressed is unique for the individual and determines his or her prakriti (physical constitution). Prakriti is said to be fixed at the time of conception, and does not change during the individual's lifetime[8]. Most people have one predominant dosha, a secondary dosha, and a small amount of the third. Some may have two dominant and a small amount of the third. It is rare for all three doshas to occur in equal amounts. Any disturbance from the natural balance of the doshas causes impairment of health. Therapies are targeted at the doshas that are imbalanced.

1.2.2 - Gunas

In addition to the tridoshas that provide the framework for the physical constitution, Ayurveda recognizes Trigunas (three qualities of the mind) that determine the psychological attitudes. The three gunas – Sattva, Rajas and Tamas – are psychological analogues to the tridoshas, and play an important role in shaping behavior[8]. Sattva is the creative influence associated with intelligence, purity and poise. Rajas is associated with passion and action. Tamas is associated with ignorance and inertia. Gunas impel people to behave in certain ways. Everyone is endowed with all three gunas, but one guna may dominate others at any given time. By observing their dominant guna(s), people can identify actions that are particularly well suited to their growth. The spiritual significance of gunas is discussed extensively in the Bhagavad Gita, the most revered Hindu scripture[9]. A proper knowledge of dosha-guna combinations can help Ayurvedic physicians deliver appropriate individualized treatment.

1.2.3 – Dhatus, Malas and Srotas

Dhatus are basic components that support the structural and functional aspects of the body. There are seven Dhatus: Rasa (plasma), Rakta (blood), Mamsa (muscle), Meda (fat), Asthi (bone), Majja (bone marrow) and Shukra (sperm or ovum). Malas are the metabolic waste products. There are three Malas: Mutra (urine), Purisha (feces) and Sweda (sweat).

According to Ayurveda, there are vast networks of channels, called Srotas, which transport air, water, food, malas, dhatus and nerve impulses within the human body. Some srotas are large, while others are minute. Large srotas and their functions as described by Charaka[10] are presented below (Table 1.2):

Srota	Transports	Srota	Transports
Pranavaha	Vital breath	Swedavaha	Sweat
Udakavaha	Water	Mootravaha	Urine
Annavaha	Food	Pureeshavaha	Fecal matter
Rasavaha	Plasma	Sukravaha	Sperm/Ovum components
Raktavaha	Blood		
Mamsavaha	Muscle components	Majjavaha	Bone Marrow components
Medovaha	Fat components	Asthivaha	Bone components

Table 1.2: Large srotas and their functions

1.2.4 – Agni, Ojas and Ama[11-15]

All of the digestive and metabolic processes of the body are under the control of Agni, which means fire in Sanskrit. There are 13 kinds of agnis, divided into three groups: one Jatharagni, five Bhutagnis and seven Dhatvagnis. Of these, jatharagni is primary. The bhutagnis and dhatvagnis continue the process started by jatharagni. It is interesting to note that in the Bhagavad Gita, Lord Krishna identifies himself with jatharagni among all the agnis in the body. He says: "Dwelling in the bodies of living beings as Vaishvanara (Jatharagni) and working with prana and apana, I digest the four kinds of food."[9]

Jatharagni operates in the mouth, stomach and intestinal regions. It transforms the ingested food into a fluid form (ahara rasa) that can be easily processed by the bhutagnis. There are five bhutagnis, one for each mahabhuta, situated in the liver. Each bhutagni transforms its corresponding mahabhuta in the ahara rasa into a suitable form for the dhatvagnis' action. There are seven dhatvagnis, each one specific to a dhatu. From the ahara rasa processed by bhutagni, the dhatvagnis synthesize materials required for their respective dhatus.

In addition to supporting the integrity and function of dhatus, agni also helps to produce Ojas, which means vigor in Sanskrit. Ojas is responsible for strength, vitality and immunity. The supreme essence of each dhatu, beginning from rasa dhatu to shukra dhatu, combines to form ojas. Charaka, the renowned Ayurvedic physician, compared the formation of ojas to the formation of honey[16]. Just as bees make honey from the essence of flowers, ojas is made from the tissue elements.

When agni is weak, it leads to incomplete digestion and metabolism of food, producing products called Ama. These products linger in the body for some time and can produce toxins that lead to disease[17].

1.2.5 – Diagnosis of Disease[18]

> A physician who fails to enter the body of a patient with the lamp of knowledge and understanding can never treat diseases.
>
> \- Charaka

Diagnosis of disease is done methodically, following a number of steps that include threefold examination (Trividha Pariksha), eightfold examination (Ashtavidha Pariksha) and tenfold examination (Dashavidha Pariksha).

Threefold examination

- Visual observation (Darshana)
- Touch (Sparshana)
- Questioning (Prashna)

Eightfold examination

- Pulse (Nadi)
- Tongue (Jihva)
- Urine (Mutra)
- Feces (Purisha)
- Physical Characteristics (Akrti)
- Eyes (Dris)
- Voice (Shabda)
- Skin (Sparasha)

Tenfold examination

- Physical constitution (Prakriti)
- Pathological state (Vikriti)
- Quality of the tissues (Sara)
- Body type (Sharira Pramana)
- Daily habits (Satmya)
- Mental constitution (Sattva)
- Digestive power (Ahara Shakti)
- Capacity for exercise (Vyayama Shakti)
- Age (Ayu)
- Quality of the body (Sharira Sanhana)

1.2.6 – Treatment of Disease[19-21]

Treatment of diseases in Ayurveda primarily consists of two types: Shodhana (cleansing) and Shamana (palliation). Shodhana is performed in three stages: Poorvakarma (preparatory procedures), Pradhanakarma (main cleansing procedures) and Paschatkarma (post procedures).

Poorvakarma prepares the body for the main cleansing processes by Dipana (kindling the digestive fire) and Pachana (facilitating the breakdown of ama), Snehana (oleation) and Swedana (sweating).

Pradhanakarma consists of five major cleansing procedures: Vamana (emesis), Virechana (purgation), Basti (enema), Nasya (nasal administration) and Raktamoksha (blood cleansing). These vital cleansing processes are also commonly referred to as Panchakarma (five therapies).

Paschatkarma is the third and final stage of shodhana karma. It helps to nourish, strengthen and balance the newly cleansed body. It consists of a proper diet regimen, appropriate physical exercise and herbal treatments.

Shamana (palliation therapy) is milder than shodhana. Shamana is used when shodhana is not appropriate due to weakness of the patient or other reasons. Shamana treatment helps to balance the doshas. There are seven types of shamana: Dipana, Pachana, Kshudha Nigraha (fasting), Trut Nigraha (minimizing consumption of water), Vyayama (exercising), Atapa seva (sunbathing) and Maruta Seva (breathing exercises).

Ayurvedic treatment is designed to meet each person's needs based on his or her constitution. The focus is primarily on restoring the doshas to their natural state. Ayurveda adopts a number of strategies to restore the sick to full health, and patients are actively involved in the healing process.

1.2.7 – Dravyaguna Vigyana[22,23]

Ayurveda uses plants, animal products and minerals as medicine. Dravyaguna Vigyana (the science of materials used as medicines) is Ayurvedic pharmacology. According to Ayurveda, every dravya (drug) is composed of panchamahabutas, just like the human body. The panchamahabhutika composition of the drug determines its action and efficacy. Appropriate medicines enhance the doshas that have become weak while simultaneously subduing the doshas that have become excessive. Medicines are chosen based on their inherent qualities such as Rasa (taste), Guna (property), Veerya (potency), Vipaka (metabolites) and Prabhava (specific action). These five are called Rasapanchaka.

1.2.7.1 – Rasa

Rasa is an important quality that can be detected by the tongue. A dravya can have more than one taste. The dominant taste is referred to as rasa and the others as anurasa. There are six rasas: Madhura (sweet), Amla (sour), Lavana (salty), Katu (pungent), Tikta (bitter) and Kashaya (astringent). The panchamahabhutika composition of rasas and their influence on doshas are summarized below (Table 1.3):

Rasa	Composition	Influence on Doshas	
		Increases	Decreases
Madhura (sweet)	Prithvi + Apo	Kapha	Vata/Pitta
Amla (sour)	Prithvi + Teja	Pitta/Kapha	Vata
Lavana (salty)	Apo + Teja	Pitta/Kapha	Vata
Katu (pungent)	Vayu + Teja	Pitta/Vata	Kapha
Tikta (bitter)	Akasha + Vayu	Vata	Kapha/Pitta
Kashaya (astrigent)	Vayu + Prithvi	Vata	Kapha/Pitta

Table 1.3: Composition of rasas and their influence on doshas

1.2.7.2 – Gurvadi Guna

Dravyas have qualities called gurvadi gunas. There are 20 gurvadi gunas (10 pairs of opposites) which are listed below (Table 1.4):

Pairs of Gurvadi Gunas	
Guru (heavy)	Laghu (light)
Manda (slow)	Tikshma (fast)
Sita (cold)	Ushna (hot)
Snigdha (uncutous)	Ruksha (non-unctous)
Slasma (smooth)	Khara (rough)
Sthira (immobile)	Sara (mobile)
Mridu (soft)	Katina (hard)
Visada (clear)	Picchila (slimy)
Sandra (solid)	Drava (liquid)
Sthula (bulky)	Sukshma (micro)

Table 1.4: Gurvadi Gunas

1.2.7.3 – Veerya

Veerya is the power that performs actions. All actions take place only because of veerya. There are two broad categories of veerya; Ushna (hot) and Sita (cold).

1.2.7.4 – Vipaka

A dravya rasa becomes Vipaka after undergoing digestion. There are three types of Vipakas: Madura (sweet), Amla (sour) and Katu (pungent). Madhura and lavana rasas form madhura vipaka, amla rasa forms amla vipaka, and katu and kashaya rasas form katu vipaka.

1.2.7.5 – Prabhava

Prabhava is defined as a specific property of a drug by virtue of which it produces a specific action that is different from another drug with the same set of rasa, guna, veerya and vipaka. For example the rasa, guna, veerya and vipaka of Danti (Baliosperum montanum) and Chitraka (Plumbgo zeylanica) are similar, but danti produces purgation and chitraka does not. The purgative action of danti is attributed to its prabhava.

1.2.8 – Major Branches of Ayurveda

Ayurveda is traditionally divided into eight major divisions:

- Kayachikitsa: Internal Medicine
- Shalyatantra: Surgery
- Salakyatantra: Ear, Nose, Throat, Ophthalmology and Dentistry
- Balatantra: Pediatrics
- Agadatantra: Toxicology
- Bhutavidya: Psychiatry
- Rasayanatantra: Geriatrics and rejuvenation
- Vijkaranatantra: Sexual function and reproduction

1.3 – Classic Ayurvedic Treatises and Brahmi

The Charaka Samhita is considered to be the first recorded treatise on Ayurveda. It was originally written by the physician Atreya (about 1000 BC) and later revised by Charaka and Drdhabala[24]. The Charaka Samhita mainly concentrates on Kayachikitsa.

The next major work was the Sushruta Samhita (1000-500 BC), written by the physician Sushruta[24]. It deals mainly with the theory and practice of surgery. One of the often quoted definitions of health comes from the Sushruta Samhita[25]:

> Sama dosha sama agnischa sama dhatu mala kriyaaha
> Prasanna atma indriya mannah swastha iti abhidheeyate

This means: One is in perfect health when the three doshas, digestive fire, all the body tissues and components, and all the excretory functions are in perfect order with a pleasantly disposed and controlled mind, senses and spirit.

The Astanga Hridaya is accepted as the third major treatise on Ayurveda. It was written by Vagbhata around 550-600 AD. It is an integration of Charaka's and Sushruta's work[26].

The Charaka Samhita, Sushruta Samhita and Astanga Hridaya are collectively known as Brihattrayi (major triad). These works on Ayurveda have extensively referred to Brahmi.

1.4 – Another Herb Called Brahmi

In some Ayurvedic literature, Centella asiatica (Gotu kola) has also been referred to as Brahmi[27,28], but Bacopa monniera and Centella asiatica are distinctly different. Taxonomically, Bacopa monniera belongs to the Scrophulariaceae family, whereas Centella asiatica belongs to Apiaceae [29]. Their dravyagunas are similar, as illustrated below (Table 1.5)[5,30]:

	B. Monniera	C. Asiatica
Rasa	Tikta, Kashaya	Tikta, Kashaya
Guna	Laghu, Snigdha, Sara	Laghu
Veerya	Sita	Sita
Vipaka	Madhura	Madhura

Table 1.5: Dravyagunas of Bacopa monniera and Centella asiatica

Both herbs enhance cognitive functions, but B. monniera is more powerful. B. monniera is used to treat major disorders such as insanity and epilepsy, whereas C. asiatica is a general rejuvenator and is even eaten as a vegetable. In ancient Sanskrit writing, B. monniera has been referred to as Jala (water) Brahmi whereas C. asiatica has been called Mandukaparni. Warrier[28] has addressed the controversy in great detail and concluded that Brahmi has to be identified as Bacopa monniera and Mandukaparni as Centella asiatica.

1.5 – Synonyms

A few synonyms of Bacopa monniera are listed below[31]:

- Bramia monniera pennel
- Moniera cuneifolia Michaux
- Herpestis monniera (L)
- Gratiola monniera L
- Lysimachia monniera L. Cent

Bacopa monniera is well known throughout India by different names, including Brahmi, Nirbrahmi, Nirubrahmi, Nirparmi, Sambrani chettu, Brihmisak, and others[28,32].

1.6 – Description, Habitat and Cultivation

Bacopa monniera is a small perennial creeping plant with a deep green color. It has numerous branches with leaves arranged on opposite sides of the creeping stem. The leaves are small, soft, thick, juicy and oval-shaped. The stem is long (10-30 cm), soft, juicy and readily forms roots at the nodes that go directly into the soil. The plant produces flowers and fruits. The solitary auxiliary flowers have five petals, and are usually pale blue, purple or white. The fruits are oval and contain numerous seeds.

The genus Bacopa includes more than 100 species of aquatic plants and is distributed throughout the warmer regions of the world. It is reported to grow in Asia, Australia and North and South America[33]. It grows abundantly throughout India in wet, damp and marshy areas such as the borders of irrigated fields, streams, water channels and tanks. It grows at lower elevations as well as at altitudes up to 4000 ft. Bacopa monniera can be easily cultivated, as it grows in a wide range of soils and climates. It thrives in poorly drained soil at temperatures between 33 to 40 °C, and at humidities between 65% to 80%[34]. Bacopa monniera can be propagated by seed, cuttings and root division. Seed propagation is not satisfactory due to frequent seedling death at the two-leaf stage[35]. The ideal planting materials are cuttings containing a few leaves, nodes and roots. The proper planting time is March-June (India). Irrigation is necessary in the absence of regular rainfall. Harvesting is done between October and November. The harvest is traditionally dried by spreading the plants under shade at room temperature. However, it has been reported that drying at 80 °C in an oven for 30 minutes followed by conventional drying enhances bacoside content compared to conventional drying alone[36]. Storing harvested material before drying considerably reduces bacoside content. Total saponin content varies by season, and the distribution of saponins is different in each part of the plant[37]. Maximum bacoside yield is obtained during August-October, with the highest content found in the leaves[38].

Bacopa monniera has the potential to accumulate toxic elements[39]. It has been reported that arsenic, cadmium, chromium, copper, iron, mercury, nickel, lead and zinc were found in naturally-grown plants located in polluted areas. Because of this, plants grown in polluted areas should not be used for medicinal purposes.

The annual demand for Brahmi was estimated at 5000 metric tons in 2008[40]. Most of the demand is currently met from natural resources. However, demand is increasing rapidly and research is being pursued to increase production.

References

1 M S Premila. Ayurvedic Herbs: a clinical guide to the healing plants of traditional Indian medicine. The Haworth Press Inc, Binghamton, NY, 2006.

2 Stefanie Schwartz. Psychoactive herbs in veterinary behavior medicine. Blackwell Publishing Ltd, Oxford UK, 2005.

3 Robert M Hackman. Antioxidants that entertain the brain. Nutrition Science News (1998) 10: 530-538.

4 P M Kidd. A review of nutrients and botanicals in the integrative management of cognitive dysfunction. Alternative Medicine Review (1999) 4(3): 144-161.

5 Gyanendra Pandey. Dravyaguna Vijnana: Vol I. Chowkhamba Krishnadas Academy, Varanasi, India, 2005.

6 Hari Sharma, H M Chandola, Gurdip Singh, Gopal Basisht. Utilization of Ayurveda in health care: an approach for prevention, health promotion and treatment of disease. Part 2 – Ayurveda in primary health care. The Journal of Alternative and Complementary Medicine (2007) 13(10): 1135-1150.

7 Hari Sharma, H M Chandola. Ayurvedic concept of obesity, metabolic syndrome and diabetes mellitus. J Altern Compl Med (2011) 17(6): 549-552.

8 S Shilpa, C G Venkatesha Murthy. Understanding personality from Ayurvedic perspective for psychological assessment: A case. Ayu (2011) 32(1): 12-19.

9 Saligrama C Subbarao. Bhagavad Gita. Translation and selected commentary. Saligrama Publishing, Newark, DE, 2010.

10 R K Sharma and Bhagwan Dash. Caraka Samhita (text with English translation and critical exposition based on Cakrapani Datta's Ayurveda Dipika) Volume 2. Chowkhamba Sanskrit Series Office, Varanasi, India, Reprint 2007.

11 Akash Kumar Agarwal, C R Yadav, M S Meena. Physiological aspects of agni. Ayu (2010) 31(3): 395-398.

12 Singh Akhilesh Kumar. A critical review on Ayurvedic concept of agnimandya (loss of appetite). JSPI (2012) 1(2): 5-8.

13 Narendra Shanker Tripathi. Concept of agni in Ayurveda. Asian Journal of Modern and Ayurvedic Medical Science (2012) 1(1): 1-5.

14 Sangeeta Gehlot, B M Singh. Concept of ojas: a scientific overview. The Indian Journal of Research Anvikshiki (2010) 2(3): 1-6.

15 Sanjeev S Tonni. Contemporary study on Ama. International Journal of Ayurvedic and Herbal Medicine (2012) 2(5): 760-765.
16 R K Sharma and Bhagwan Dash. Caraka Samhita (text with English translation and critical exposition based on Cakrapani Datta's Ayurveda Dipika) volume 1. Chowkhamba Sanskrit Series Office, Varanasi, India, Reprint 2007.
17 R K Sharma and Bhagwan Dash. Caraka Samhita (text with English translation and critical exposition based on Cakrapani Datta's Ayurveda Dipika) volume 4. Chowkhamba Sanskrit Series Office, Varanasi, India, Reprint 2007.
18 Anne McIntyre. Herbal treatment of children: western and Ayurvedic perspectives. Elsevier Butterworth-Heinemann, New York, 2005.
19 Todd Caldecott. Ayurveda: the divine science of life. Mosby Elsevier, Philadelphia, 2006.
20 Lakshmi Chandra Mishra. "Health care and disease management" in Scientific Basis for Ayurvedic Therapies. Edited by Lakshmi Chandra Mishra. CRC Press, Boca Raton, FL, 2004.
21 Ajay Kumar Sharma. "Panchakarma therapy in Ayurvedic medicine" in Scientific Basis for Ayurveda Therapies. Edited by Lakshmi Chandra Mishra, CRC Press, Boca Raton, FL, 2004.
22 Priya Vart Sharma. Essentials of Ayurveda, text and translation of sodasangahrdayam. Motilal Banarsidass Publishers, Delhi, Reprint 2009.
23 Sudipt Kumar Rath, Ashashri Shinde, Lalit Nagar, Ringzin Lamo, Pankaj Gahunge, Naresh Kumar Khemani. Prabhava revisited. International Journal of Ayurvedic and Herbal Medicine (2012) 2(3): 569-573.
24 Bala V Manyam. Dementia in Ayurveda. The Journal of Alternative and Complementary Medicine (1999) 5(1): 81-88.
25 K. R. Srikantha Murthy. Illustrated Susruta Samhita (text, English translation, notes, appendices and indices) Vol I. Chaukhambha Orientalia, Varanasi, India, fourth edition 2010.
26 K R Srikantha Murthy. Vagbhata's Astanga Hrdayam (text, English translation, notes, appendices and indices). Chowkhamba Krishnadas Academy, Varanasi, India, seventh edition, 2010.
27 K R Srikantha Murthy. Bhavaprakasa of Bhavamisra (text, English translation, notes, appendices and index) Volume 1. Chowkhamba Krishnadas Academy, Varanasi, India, reprinted 2008.
28 P K Warrier, V P K Nambiar and C Ramani Kutty. Indian medicinal plants. Vol 1. Orient Longman, Hyderabad, India, reprinted 2005.
29 Manisha N Trivedi, Archana Khemani, Urmila D Vachhani, Charmi P Shah, D D Santani. Comparative pharmacognostic and phytochemical investigation of two plant species valued as medhya rasayanas. International Journal of Applied Biology and Pharmaceutical Technology (2011) 2(3): 28-34.
30 Gyanendra Pandey. Dravyaguna Vijnana: Vol II. Chowkhamba Krishnadas Academy, Varanasi, India, 2005.
31 M Rajani. "Bacopa Monnieri, a Nootropic Drug" in Bioactive Molecules and Medicinal Plants, Edited by K G Ramawat and J M Merillon, Springer, 2008.
32 E R B Shanmugasundaram, G K Mohammed Akbar, K Radha

Shanmugasundaram. Brahmighritham, an Ayurvedic herbal formula for the control of epilepsy. Journal of Ethnopharmacology (1991) 33: 269-276.

33 Shalini Mathur, Srikant Sharma, M M Gupta, Sushil Kumar. Evaluation of an Indian germplasm collection of the medicinal plant Bacopa monnieri (L.) pennell by use of multivariate approaches. Euphytica (2003) 133: 255-265.

34 NIIR Board of Consultants. The Complete Book On Jatropha (Bio-Diesel) with Ashwagandha, Stevia, Brahmi & Jatamansi Herbs (cultivation, processing & uses). Asia Pacific Business Press, 2006.

35 A Parale, R Barmukh, T Nikam. Influence of organic supplements on production of shoot and callus biomass and accumulation of bacoside in Bacopa monniera (L.) pennell. Physiol Mol Biol Plants (2010) 16(2): 167-175.

36 A P Gupta, S Mathur, M M Gupta, Sushil Kumar. Effect of the method of drying on the bacoside-A content of the harvested Bacopa monniera shoots revealed using a high performance thin layer chromatography method. Journal of Medicinal and Aromatic Plant Sciences (1998) 20: 1052-1055.

37 W Phrompittayarat, K Jetiyanon, S Wittaya-Areekul, W Putalun, H Tanaka, I Khan, K Ingkaninan. Influence of seasons, different plant parts, and plant growth stages on saponin quantity and distribution in Bacopa monnieri. SJST (2011) 33(2): 193-199.

38 M Sharma, R K Khajuria, S Mallubhotla. Annual variation in bacoside content of Bacopa monnieri (L.) wettst plants. IJPBS (2013) 4(4): 266-271.

39 K Hussain, A K Abdussalam, C P Ratheesh, S Nabeesa. Heavy metal accumulation potential and medicinal property of Bacopa monnieri – a paradox. Journal of Stress Physiology and Biochemistry (2011) 7(4): 39-50.

40 Gayle Engels, Josef Brinckmann. Bacopa. HerbalGram: The Journal of the American Botanical Council (2011) 91: 1-4.

2 – Constituents and Analysis

2.1 – Constituents

Bacopa monniera has versatile healing powers because it contains a unique mixture of bioactive components. During the last eight decades, a number of these components - including alkaloids, flavonoids, saponins and sterols - have been isolated and characterized[1,2,3]. Major compounds of pharmacological interest are dammarane-type triterpenoidal saponins with either a jujubogenin or a pseudojujubogenin as an aglycone. In addition, a number of phenylethanoid glycosides and other glycosides, including cucurbitacins have been reported. Several compounds found in Brahmi are presented below in Table 2.1 and most of their structures are shown in Table 2.2.

Initial investigations reported the presence of two saponins (designated as bacosides A and B) in the alcoholic extract of the plant, to which the nootropic activities of Brahmi were attributed[38,39]. Bacosides A and B were found to have the same aglycone and carbohydrate moieties. They differed in optical rotation: bacoside A was levorotary, whereas bacoside B was dextrorotary. This was attributed to differences in the configuration of the carbohydrate chain in the two saponins[40]. Since the pharmacological properties of Brahmi were mainly attributed to bacosides A and B, they were considered bioactive markers of Brahmi. Most published studies on Brahmi extracts refer to bacoside content, and nutraceutical formulations of Brahmi are marketed with label claims of bacoside content. Recently, it has been discovered that bacosides A and B are not single chemical entities, but rather mixtures of four triglycosidic and four diglycosidic saponins, respectively[13,41]. Bacoside A is a mixture of bacoside A3, bacopaside II, bacopaside X, and bacopasaponin C, and bacoside B is a mixture of bacopaside N1, bacopaside N2, bacopaside IV and bacopaside V.

Compound	Reference	Compound	Reference
Bacoside A_1	4	Bacopasaponin A Bacopasaponin B Bacopasaponin C	15
Bacoside A_2	5		
Bacoside A_3	6	Bacopasaponin D	16
Bacoside A_4 Bacoside A_5	7	Bacopasaponin E Bacopasaponin F	17
Bacoside A_6	21	Bacopasaponin H	18
Bacopaside I Bacosapide II	8	Bacopasaponin G Bacopaside A Bacopaside B Bacopaside C	9
Bacosapide III	9		
Bacospaside IV Bacopaside V	10	Bacobitacin A Bacobitacin B Bacobitacin C Bacobitacin D	20
Bacopaside VI Bacopaside VII Bacopaside VIII	11	Cucurbitacin E	20,32
Bacopaside IX	12	Bacopaside N1 Bacopaside N2	13
Bacopaside X	13	Brahmine	22
Bacopaside XI Bacopaside XII	14	Nicotine	23,33
		Herpestine	23
Monnieraside I Monnieraside II Monnieraside III Plantainoside B	19	Bacosterol	25
		Bacosine	25,2
		Bacosterol-3-O-ß-D-glucopyranoside Luteolin-7-O-ß-glucopyroniside	25
Betulinic acid	27,28	Luteolin	26,34
Stigmasterol	27,29	Quercetin	26,35
Stigmastanol	27,30	Apigenin	26,36
ß-Sistosterol	27,31	D-Mannitol Hersaponin	24,37

Table 2.1: Compounds present in Brahmi

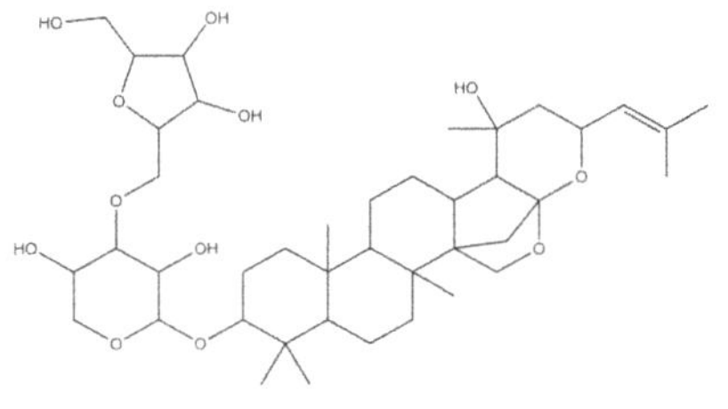

Bacoside A_1	Bacoside A_2
Bacoside A_3	Bacoside A_4
Bacoside A_5	Bacopaside I
Bacopaside II	Bacopaside III

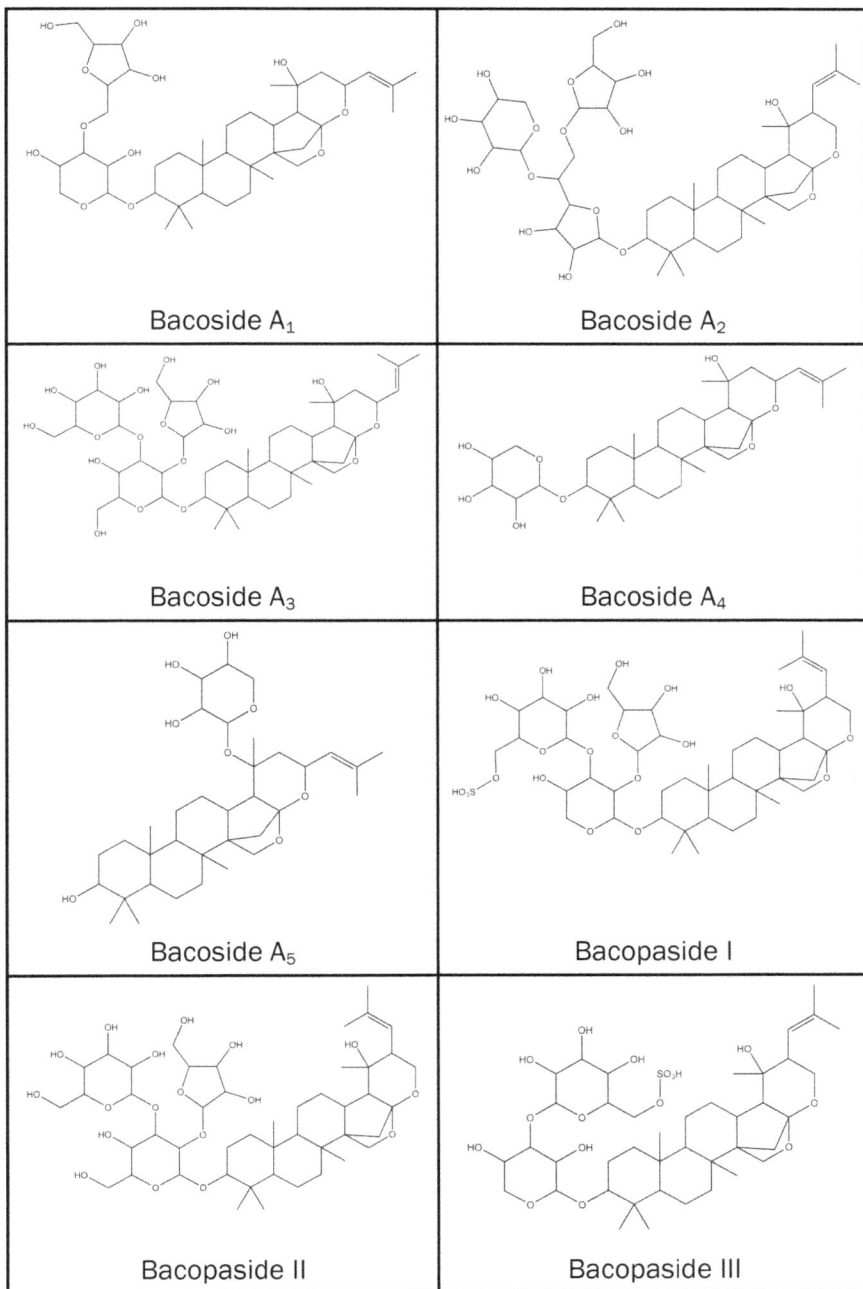

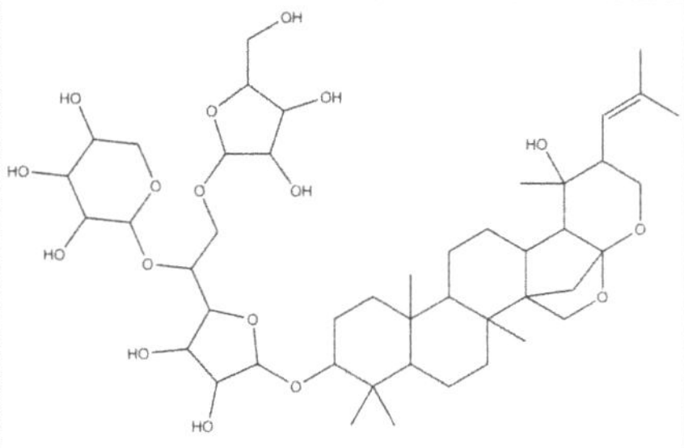

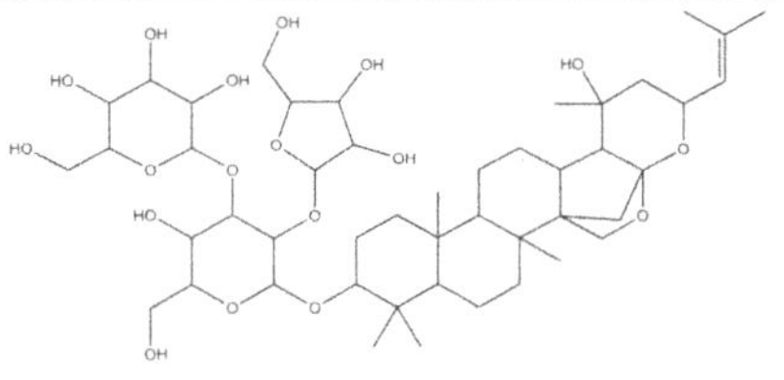

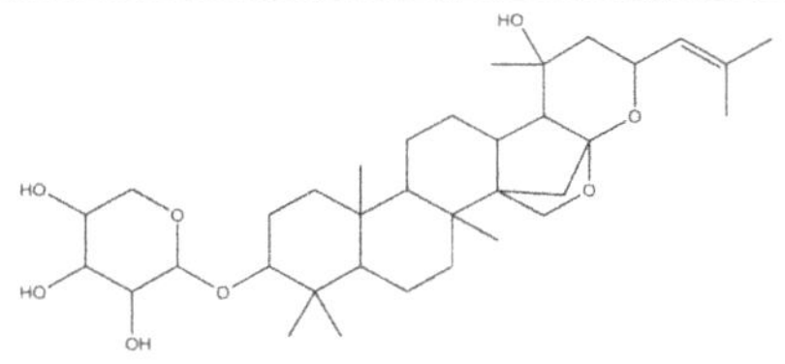

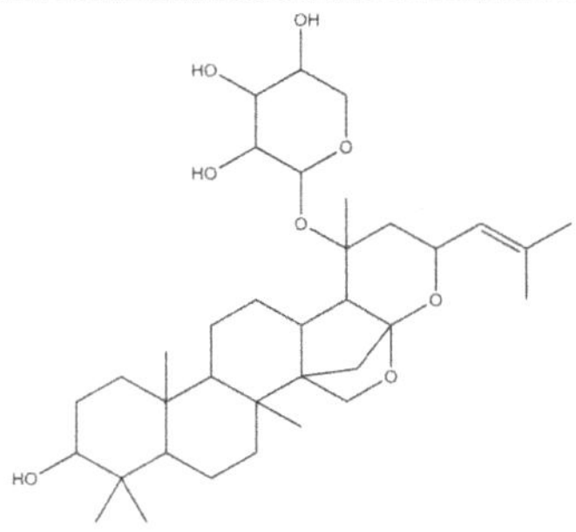

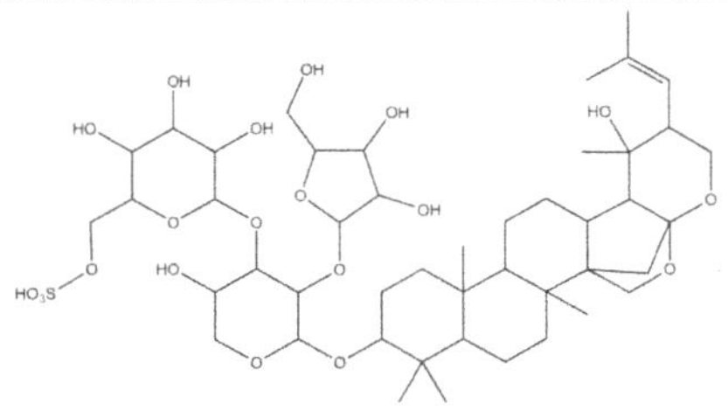

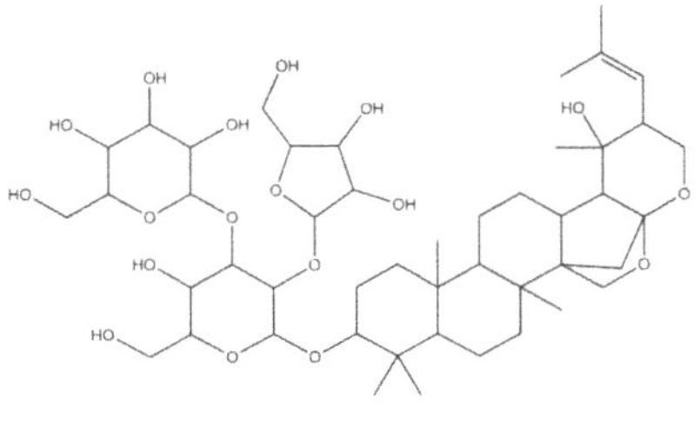

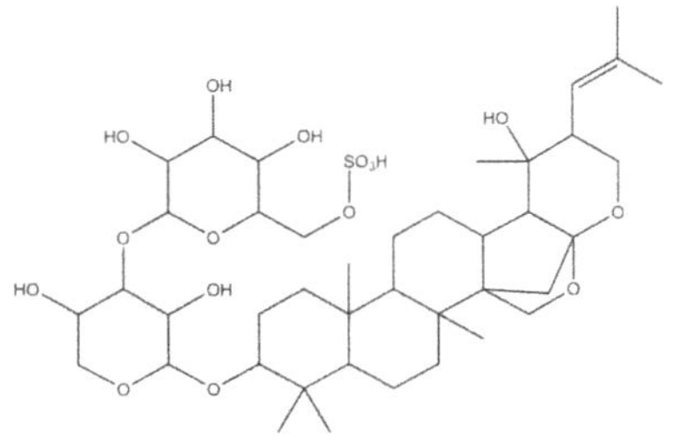

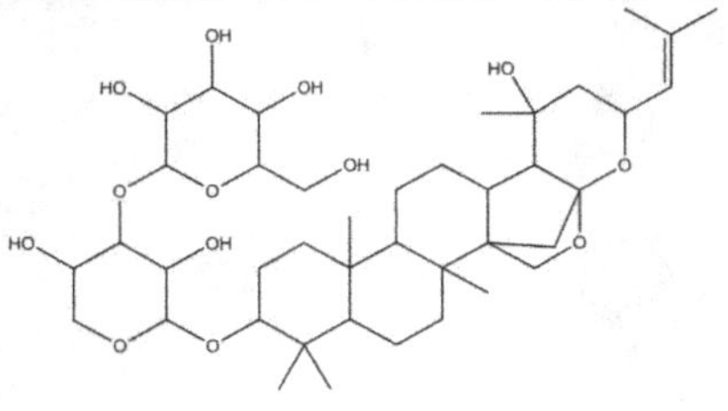

Bacopaside IV	Bacopaside V
Bacopaside VI	Bacopaside VII
Bacopaside VIII	Bacopaside IX
Bacopaside X	Bacopaside XI

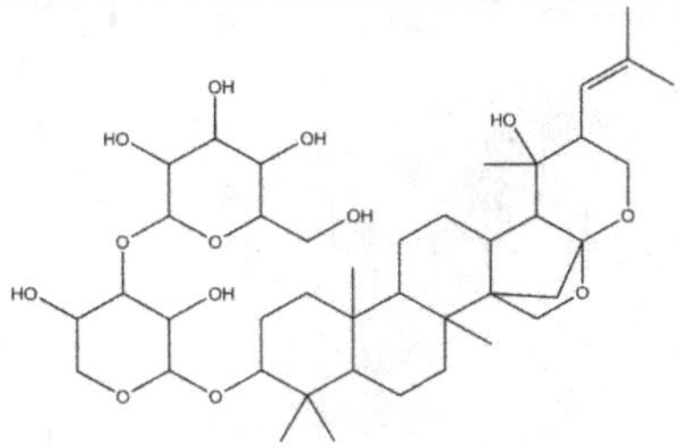

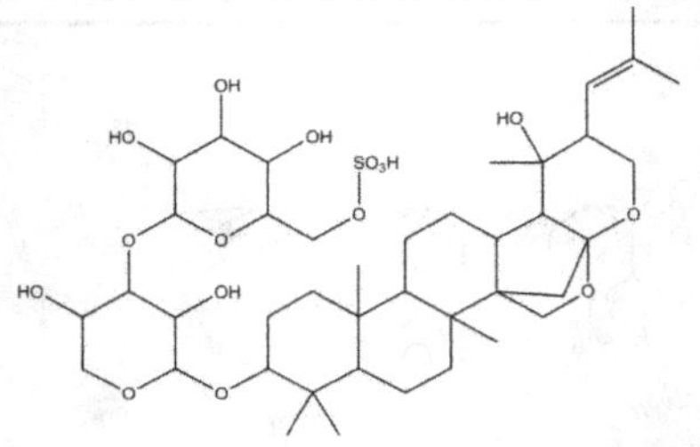

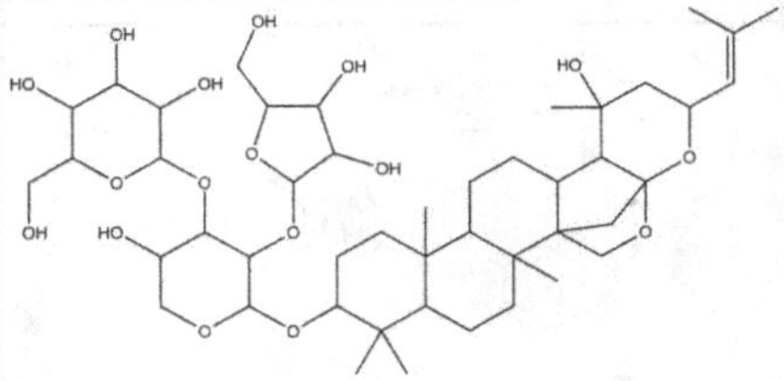

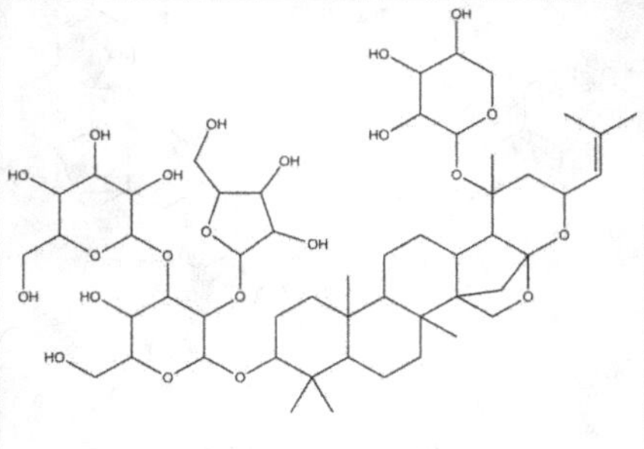

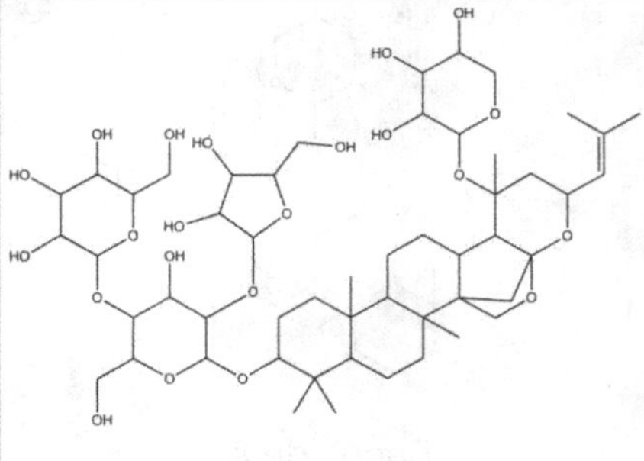

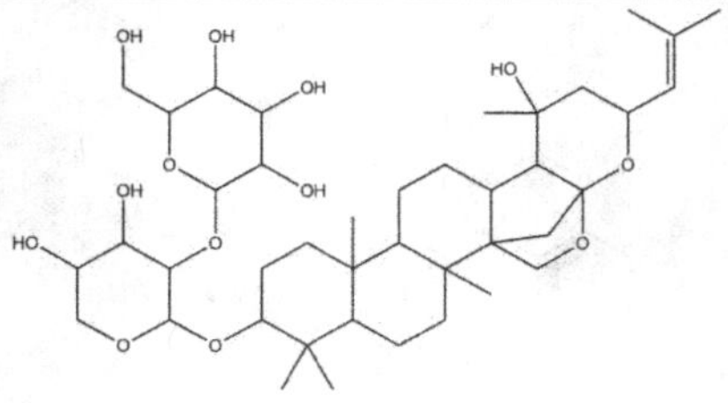

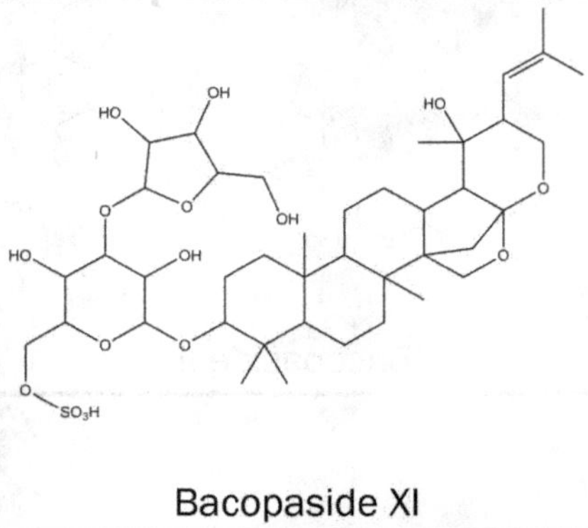

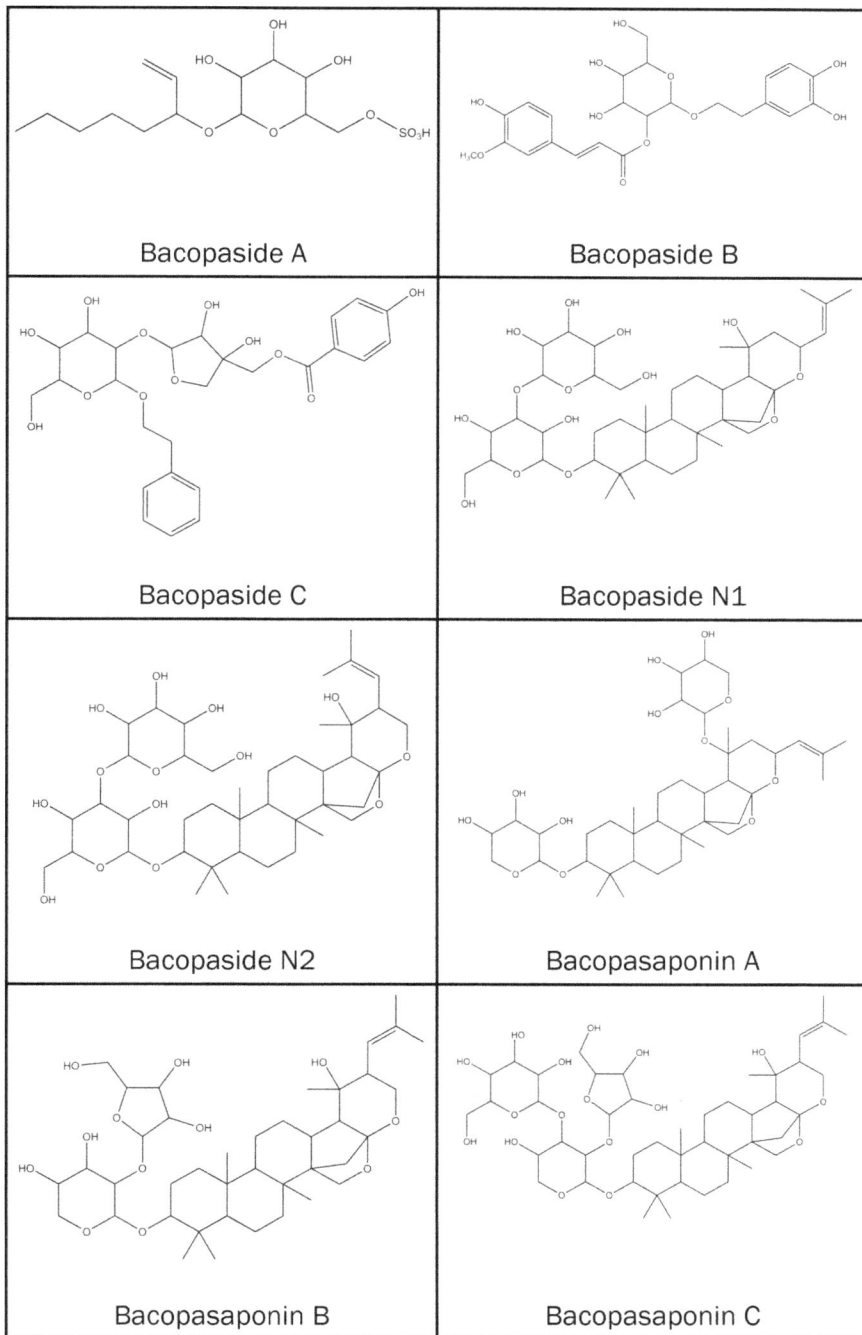

Bacopaside A	Bacopaside B
Bacopaside C	Bacopaside N1
Bacopaside N2	Bacopasaponin A
Bacopasaponin B	Bacopasaponin C

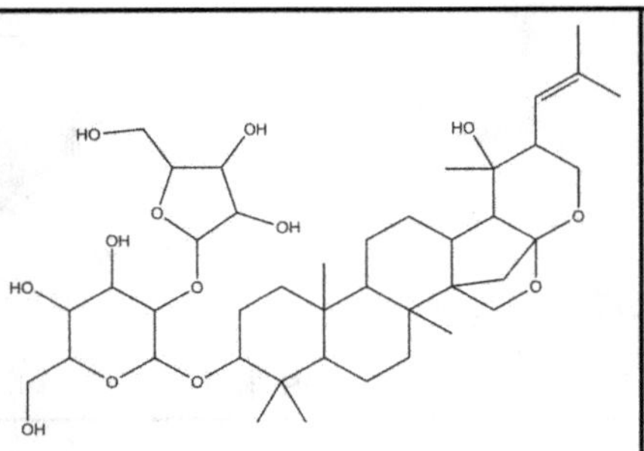

Bacopasaponin D	Bacopasaponin E
Bacopasaponin F	Bacopasaponin G
Bacopasaponin H	Cucurbitacin E

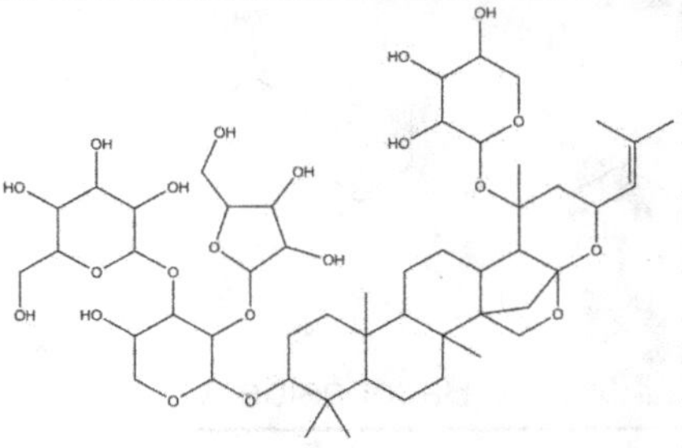

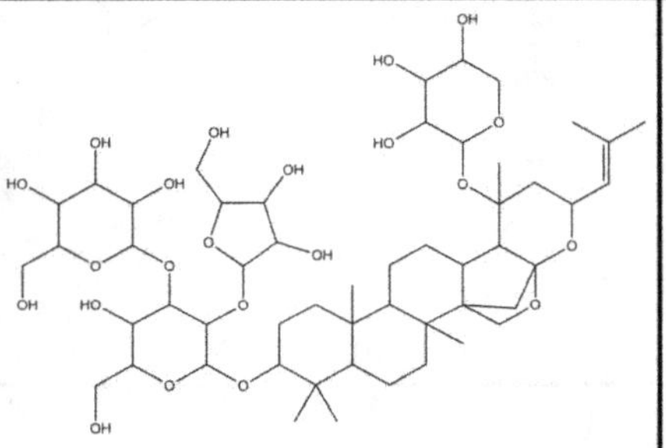

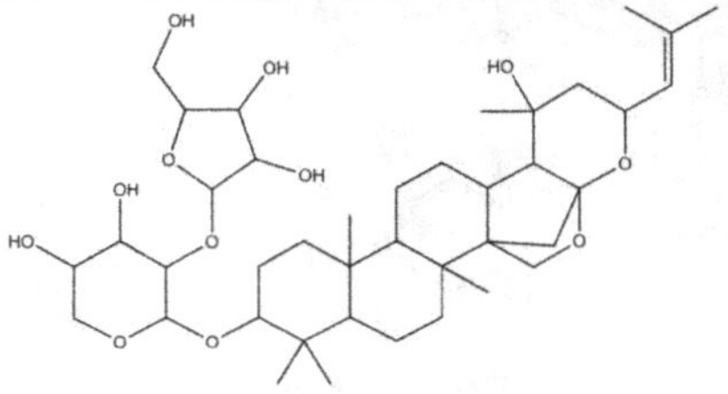

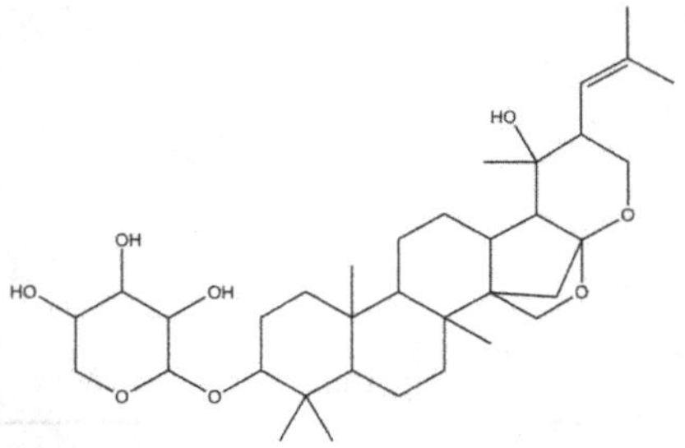

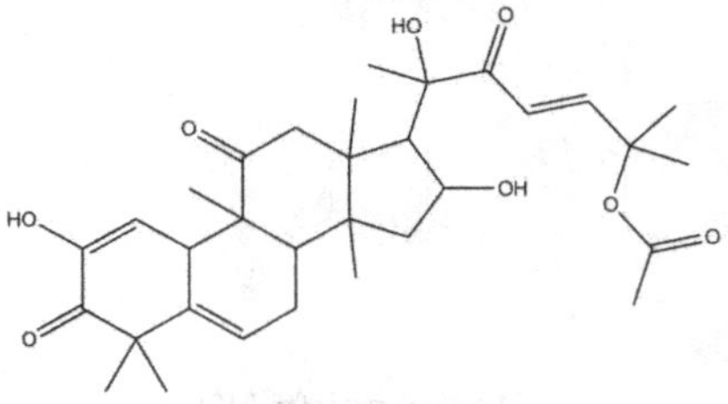

Bacobitacin A	Bacobitacin B
Bacobitacin C	Bacobitacin D
Bacosine	Bacosterol-3-O-ß-D-glucopyranoside

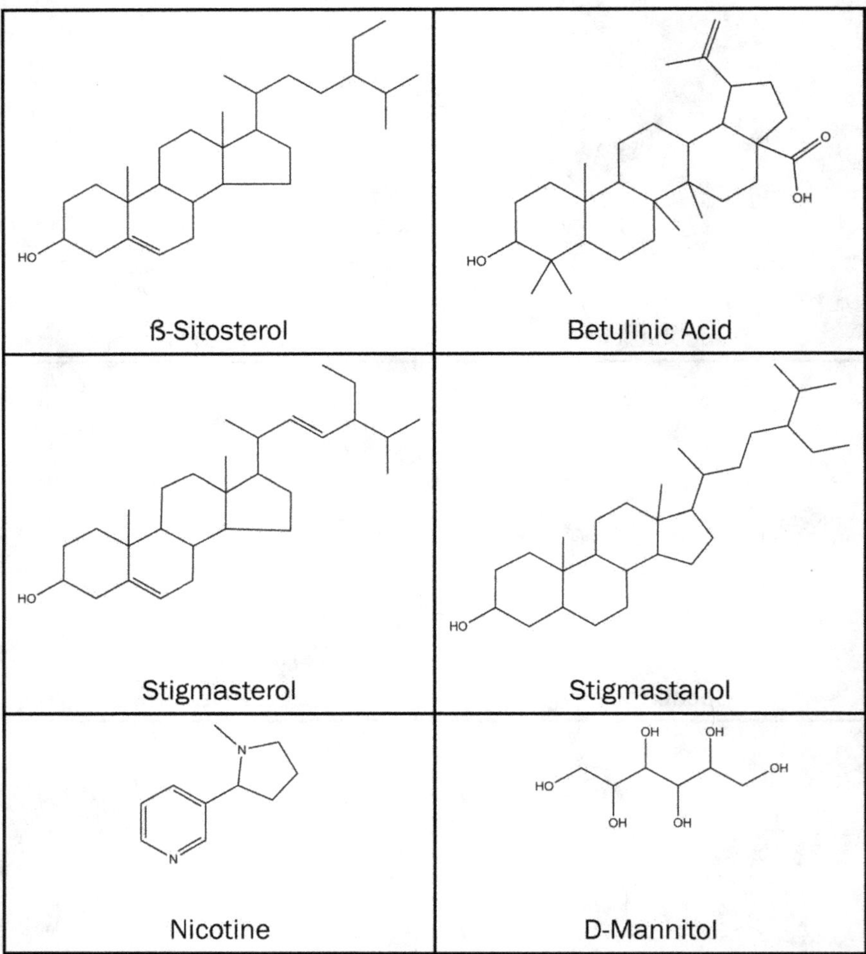
HO
ß-Sitosterol
HO
O
OH
Betulinic Acid
HO
Stigmasterol
HO
Stigmastanol
N
N
Nicotine
OH
OH
HO
OH
OH
OH
D-Mannitol

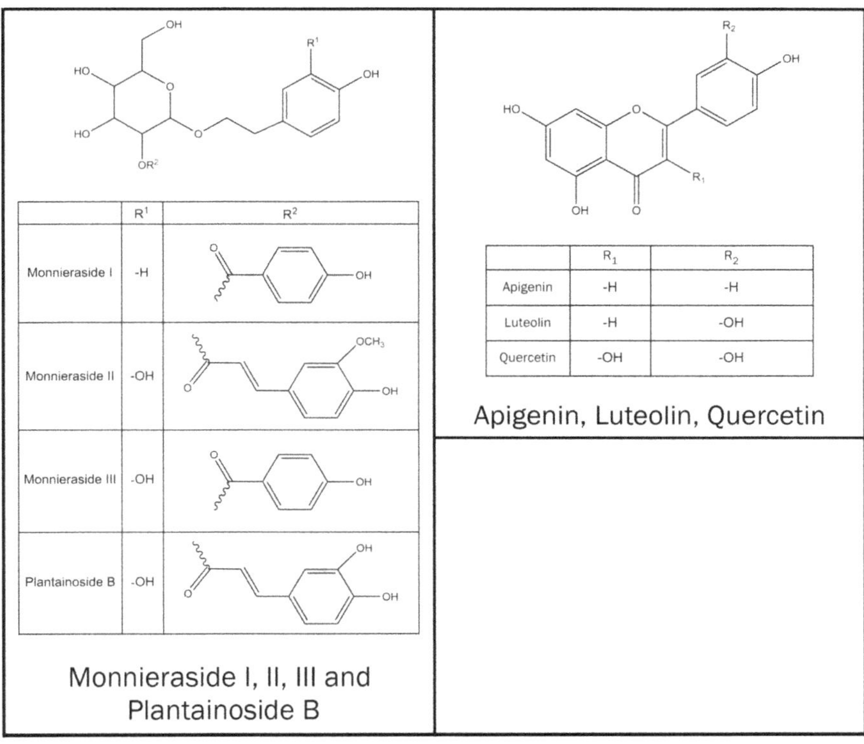

	R1	R2
Monnieraside I	-H	
Monnieraside II	-OH	
Monnieraside III	-OH	
Plantainoside B	-OH	

Monnieraside I, II, III and Plantainoside B

	R1	R2
Apigenin	-H	-H
Luteolin	-H	-OH
Quercetin	-OH	-OH

Apigenin, Luteolin, Quercetin

Table 2.2: Structures of selected compounds found in Brahmi

2.2 - Essential Nutrient Elements

Garg and coworkers[42] used neutron activation analysis to determine the elemental composition of raw Brahmi, as well as Brahmi extracted with water, methanol and methanol-water. Raw Brahmi was found to be rich in calcium, iron, potassium, chromium, manganese, copper and zinc. These essential nutrients are required for a number of biochemical processes in the body. The methanol-water extract showed comparatively higher contents of manganese, cobalt and zinc.

2.3 - Quantitation of Major Components

A number of techniques have been reported for the quantitation of Bacopa monniera, including spectrophotometry, high performance liquid chromatography (HPLC), high performance thin layer chromatography (HPTLC), supercritical fluid chromatography (SFC) and enzyme linked immunosorbent assay (ELISA).

2.3.1 – Spectrophotometry

Pal and Serin[43] reported a spectrophotometric method for the quantitative determination of total bacoside content in Bacopa monniera. The acid hydrolysis of bacosides A and B produces ebelin lactone, a conjugated triene system. The formation of ebelin lactone is quantitative and has a UV absorbance at 278 nm. Hydrolysis was conducted with 2 M sulfuric acid and the product was extracted with chloroform. The extract was evaporated to dryness under reduced pressure and the residue was dissolved in methanol, diluted appropriately. Absorbance was measured at 278 nm. Hydrolyzed bacoside A was shown to have a linear range of 5 to 50 µg/mL.

This method is used for the quality control of raw materials, but it lacks specificity, and other hydrolyzed compounds can cause interference[49].

2.3.2 – Reversed phase HPLC

Reversed phase HPLC has become the standard technique for the analysis of Bacopa monniera and its formulations. Since the major saponins found in Bacopa monniera are structurally similar, analysis is a real challenge, requiring meticulous optimization of all the relevant parameters such as stationary phase, mobile phase, flow rate, temperature, etc[44]. Furthermore, these compounds possess weak chromophores that can only be detected at wavelengths close to 200 nm. Several reversed phase HPLC methods have been reported for the separation and quantitation of Bacopa monniera components during a single run. Most of the methods used a C18 column with a PDA detector[13,41,49,45,46]. One study described the separation of major saponins within 30 minutes using a C8 column[44]. The use of a silica-based monolithic column with an evaporative light-scattering detector was reported for the simultaneous quantitation of bacosides and apigenin[47]. A micro analytical technique for screening a large number of Bacopa monniera samples using small quantities of plant materials (as little as 2 mg) was also reported[48]. HPLC-ESI-MS was used to confirm the presence of analytes from Bacopa monniera[44]. Another report described the estimation of active compounds from crude Bacopa monniera extracts using HPLC-NMR, HPLC-MS and bioassay methods[50]. A summary of results from select publications is presented in Table 2.3:

<table>
<tr><td>Column</td><td colspan="3">Shim pack Prep ODS (H) Kit Column (250 x 4.6 mm, 5 μm)</td></tr>
<tr><td>Mobile Phase</td><td colspan="3">A: Acetonitrile; B: Water with 0.05% Orthophosphoric acid</td></tr>
<tr><td>Gradient</td><td colspan="3">30% to 40% A in 25 min; 40% to 60% A in 10 min</td></tr>
<tr><td>Flow Rate</td><td>1.5 mL/min</td><td rowspan="3">Compounds analyzed</td><td rowspan="3">C1) Bacoside A_3
C2) Bacopaside II
C3) Bacopaside X
C4) Bacopasaponin C
C5) Luteolin
C6) Apigenin</td></tr>
<tr><td>Injection Volume</td><td>20 μL</td></tr>
<tr><td>Detection Wavelength</td><td>205 nm</td></tr>
<tr><td>Validation Parameters</td><td colspan="3">Linearity Range: 2-64 μg (C1-C4)
r^2: > 0.999 (C1-C4)
RSD: < 4% for all concentrations (C1-C4)
Recovery: Greater than 90% (C1-C4)</td></tr>
<tr><td>Reference</td><td colspan="3">41</td></tr>
</table>

<table>
<tr><td>Column</td><td colspan="3">Phenomenex Luna C8 (100 x 4.6 mm, 3 μm)</td></tr>
<tr><td>Mobile Phase</td><td colspan="3">A: Water; B: Methanol</td></tr>
<tr><td>Elution Method</td><td colspan="3">57% to 65% B in 30 min</td></tr>
<tr><td>Flow Rate</td><td>0.5 mL/min</td><td rowspan="4">Compounds Analyzed</td><td rowspan="4">C1) Bacoside A_3
C2) Bacopaside II
C3) Bacopasaponin C
C4) Bacopaside I
C5) Bacopaside IV
C6) Bacopaside V</td></tr>
<tr><td>Temperature</td><td>40 °C</td></tr>
<tr><td>Injection Volume</td><td>10 μL</td></tr>
<tr><td>Detection Wavelength</td><td>205 nm</td></tr>
<tr><td>Validation Parameters</td><td colspan="3">Linearity Range: 15.6-1000 μg/mL
r^2: 0.9989-0.9999
LOD: 7.2-8.8 μg/mL
Recovery: 97.0%-102.6%
Intra-day and Inter-day Variation: < 8.2%</td></tr>
<tr><td>Reference</td><td colspan="3">44</td></tr>
</table>

<table>
<tr><td>Column</td><td colspan="3">Phenomenex Luna C18 (150 x 4.6 mm, 5 μm)</td></tr>
<tr><td>Mobile Phase</td><td colspan="3">A: 0.2 M Phosphoric acid, pH 3; B: Acetonitrile</td></tr>
<tr><td>Elution Method</td><td colspan="3">Isocratic; 65% A: 35% B</td></tr>
<tr><td>Flow Rate</td><td>1 mL/min</td><td rowspan="3">Compounds Analyzed</td><td rowspan="3">C1) Bacoside A_3
C2) Bacopaside II
C3) Bacopaside X
C4) Bacopasaponin C
C5) Bacopaside I</td></tr>
<tr><td>Injection Volume</td><td>20 μL</td></tr>
<tr><td>Detection Wavelength</td><td>205 nm</td></tr>
<tr><td>Validation Parameters</td><td colspan="3">Linearity Range: 7.8-500 μg/mL
r^2: 0.9998-0.9999
LOD: 0.31-0.62 μg/mL
RSD: < 4% intra-day, < 10% inter-day
Recovery: 85.75%-103.05%</td></tr>
<tr><td>Reference</td><td colspan="3">45</td></tr>
</table>

<table>
<tr><td>Column</td><td colspan="3">Merck C18 (250 x 4 mm, 5 μm)</td></tr>
<tr><td>Mobile Phase</td><td colspan="3">A: Acetonitrile; B: Water</td></tr>
<tr><td>Elution Method</td><td colspan="3">Isocratic: 40% A: 60% B</td></tr>
<tr><td>Flow Rate</td><td>1 mL/min</td><td rowspan="4">Compound Analyzed</td><td rowspan="4">Bacoside A_3</td></tr>
<tr><td>Temperature</td><td>27 °C</td></tr>
<tr><td>Injection Volume</td><td>10 μL</td></tr>
<tr><td>Detection Wavelength</td><td>215 nm</td></tr>
<tr><td>Validation Parameters</td><td colspan="3">Linearity Range: 26-260 μg/mL
r^2: 0.9953
Intra-day RSD: < 6%
LOQ: 26 μg/mL</td></tr>
<tr><td>Reference</td><td colspan="3">46</td></tr>
</table>

<table>
<tr><th>Column</th><td colspan="3">Chromolith RP-18 (100 x 4.6 mm)</td></tr>
<tr><th>Mobile Phase</th><td colspan="3">A: Acetonitrile; B: Water</td></tr>
<tr><th>Elution Method</th><td colspan="3">Isocratic: 30% A: 70% B</td></tr>
<tr><th>Flow Rate</th><td>0.7 mL/min</td><th rowspan="4">Compounds Analyzed</th><td rowspan="4">C1) Bacopaside I
C2) Bacoside A_3
C3) Bacopaside II
C4) Bacopaside X
C5) Bacopasaponin C
C6) Apigenin</td></tr>
<tr><th>Column Temperature</th><td>25 °C</td></tr>
<tr><th>Drift Tube Temperature</th><td>95 °C</td></tr>
<tr><th>Nitrogen Flow Rate</th><td>2 L/min</td></tr>
<tr><th>Validation Parameters</th><td colspan="3">Linearity Range: 50-300 μg/mL (C1)
r^2: > 0.9970 (C5) to 0.9998 (C4)
LOD: 0.54–6.06 μg/mL
LOQ: 1.61–18.78 μg/mL
Recovery Rate: 95.8%-99.0%</td></tr>
<tr><th>Reference</th><td colspan="3">47</td></tr>
</table>

<table>
<tr><th>Column</th><td colspan="3">E Merck Chromolith RP-18e (100 x 4.6 mm)</td></tr>
<tr><th>Mobile Phase</th><td colspan="3">A: Acetonitrile; B: Water</td></tr>
<tr><th>Elution Method</th><td colspan="3">Isocratic; 30% A: 70% B</td></tr>
<tr><th>Flow Rate</th><td>0.8 mL/min</td><th rowspan="4">Compound Analyzed</th><td rowspan="4">Bacoside A</td></tr>
<tr><th>Temperature</th><td>21 °C</td></tr>
<tr><th>Injection Volume</th><td>20 μL</td></tr>
<tr><th>Detection Wavelength</th><td>205 nm</td></tr>
<tr><th>Validation Parameters</th><td colspan="3">Linearity Range: 7.8-500 μg/mL
r: 0.9999
LOD: 4 μg
LOQ: 7.8 μg
Recovery: 97.0%</td></tr>
<tr><th>Reference</th><td colspan="3">48</td></tr>
</table>

<table>
<tr><th>Column</th><td colspan="3">Phenomenex Luna C18 (250 x 4.6 mm, 5 μm)</td></tr>
<tr><th>Mobile Phase</th><td colspan="3">A: Water with 0.05 M sodium sulfate buffer, pH 2.3
B: Acetonitrile</td></tr>
<tr><th>Elution Method</th><td colspan="3">Isocratic; 68.5% A: 31.5% B</td></tr>
<tr><th>Flow Rate</th><td>1 mL/min</td><th rowspan="4">Compounds Analyzed</th><td rowspan="4">C1) Bacopasaponin F
C2) Bacopasaponin E
C3) Bacoside A_3
C4) Bacopaside II
C5) Bacopaside I
C6) Bacopaside X
C7) Bacopasaponin C
C8) Bacopaside N1
C9) Bacopaside N2
C10) Bacopaside III
C11) Bacopaside IV
C12) Bacopaside V</td></tr>
<tr><th>Temperature</th><td>30 °C</td></tr>
<tr><th>Injection Volume</th><td>20 μL</td></tr>
<tr><th>Detection Wavelength</th><td>205 nm</td></tr>
<tr><th>Validation Parameters</th><td colspan="3">Linearity Range: 20-60 μg/20 μL (C1)
r^2: 0.9939-0.9999
LOD: 0.01-0.04 μg/20 μL
LOQ: 0.03-0.124 μg/20 μL
Recovery: 94.06%-100.86%</td></tr>
<tr><th>Reference</th><td colspan="3">49</td></tr>
</table>

Table 2.3: Summary of HPLC results of Bacopa monniera from selected publications

2.3.3 – High Performance Thin Layer Chromatography (HPTLC)

HPTLC is an advanced form of conventional thin layer chromatography (TLC)[51]. It has emerged as a major analytical tool with a wide range of applications. It is used in the analysis of pharmaceuticals, herbal medicines, dietary supplements, biological and clinical samples, foods and beverages, environmental pollutants and other chemicals[52]. It provides a detailed fingerprint of the sample, making it highly attractive for the analysis of complex materials. HPTLC can be used for quantitative analysis as well as to obtain structural information on separated compounds. UV, diode-array, fluorescence spectroscopy, mass spectrometry, Fourier-transform infrared (FT-IR) and Raman spectroscopy have all been applied for the in situ determination of analytes on TLC plates[53]. Key features of HPTLC include the following[54,55]:

- Simplicity, speed and cost effectiveness

- Minimum sample clean-up
- High sample throughput
- Simultaneous processing of sample and standards
- Minimum consumption of organic solvents and minimum waste production
- No interferences from previous analyses
- Reproducibility, accuracy, reliability and robustness

A number of reports have been published on the use of HPTLC in the analysis of Bacopa monniera and its formulations. Results from select publications are summarized in Table 2.4:

Stationary Phase	RP-18 F_{254} pre-coated TLC		
Mobile Phase	Dual run; 70% Water with 5% Formic acid:30% Methanol and 50% Water with 5% Formic acid:50% Methanol		
Solvent Front Migration	90 mm	**Compounds Analyzed**	C1) Apigenin C2) Quercetin C3) Luteolin
Detection Scan	280 nm		
Validation Parameters	**Linearity Range:** 150-800 ng (C1) 200-1000 ng (C2 and C3) **r:** 0.999 **LOD:** 30 ng (C1); 40 ng (C2); 40 ng (C3) **LOQ:** 166.66 ng (C1); 200 ng (C2); 200 ng (C3) **Recovery:** 97.9%–99.8%		
Reference	26		

<table>
<tr><td>Stationary Phase</td><td colspan="4">Aluminum backed HPTLC plates coated with RP-18F_{254} silica gel</td></tr>
<tr><td>Mobile Phase</td><td colspan="4">Toluene:Methanol:Ethyl acetate (7.5:2.5:2.0)</td></tr>
<tr><td>Relative Humidity</td><td>60%</td><td rowspan="3">Compounds Analyzed</td><td colspan="2" rowspan="3">C1) Bacoside A_3
C2) Bacopaside II</td></tr>
<tr><td>Solvent Front Migration</td><td>9 cm</td></tr>
<tr><td>Detection Scan</td><td>344 nm</td></tr>
<tr><td rowspan="8">Validation Parameters</td><td colspan="2"></td><td>C1</td><td>C2</td></tr>
<tr><td colspan="2">Linearity Range (µg/spot)</td><td>5.0 - 75</td><td>5.0 - 80</td></tr>
<tr><td colspan="2">r^2</td><td>0.9989</td><td>0.9980</td></tr>
<tr><td colspan="2">LOD</td><td>0.5 µg</td><td>0.70 µg</td></tr>
<tr><td colspan="2">LOQ</td><td>0.8 µg</td><td>1.0 µg</td></tr>
<tr><td colspan="2">Inter-day Variation</td><td>1.73%</td><td>1.97%</td></tr>
<tr><td colspan="2">Intra-day Variation</td><td>1.31%</td><td>1.64%</td></tr>
<tr><td colspan="2">Recovery</td><td>98.46%</td><td>98.12%</td></tr>
<tr><td>Reference</td><td colspan="4">55</td></tr>
</table>

<table>
<tr><td>Stationary Phase</td><td colspan="3">TLC aluminum plate pre-coated with silica gel GF_{254}</td></tr>
<tr><td>Mobile Phase</td><td colspan="3">n-Butanol:Acetic acid:Water (36:6:8)</td></tr>
<tr><td>Solvent Front Migration</td><td>80 mm</td><td rowspan="2">Compound Analyzed</td><td rowspan="2">Bacoside A</td></tr>
<tr><td>Detection Scan</td><td>580 nm</td></tr>
<tr><td>Validation Parameters</td><td colspan="3">Linearity Range: 200-1200 ng
r: 0.998
LOD: 46 ng
LOQ: 139.4 ng
Recovery: 91.92% - 97.96%</td></tr>
<tr><td>Reference</td><td colspan="3">56</td></tr>
</table>

Stationary Phase	Silica gel 60 F_{254}, pre-coated TLC plates		
Mobile Phase	Ethyl Acetate:Methyl alcohol:Water (60:14:10)		
Temperature	20 °C	**Compound Analyzed**	Bacoside A
Relative Humidity	50%		
Sample Volume	5 μL		
Solvent Front Migration	8 cm		
Detection Scan	620 nm and 430 nm dual absorption-reflection mode		
Validation Parameters	**Linearity Range:** 1-20 μg **r:** 0.99 **Recovery:** 98%		
Reference	57		

Stationary Phase	Silica gel G60 F_{254}, pre-coated TLC plates		
Mobile Phase	Chloroform:Methanol:Water (18:9:0.6)		
Sample Volume	2 μL	**Compound Analyzed**	Bacoside A
Solvent Front Migration	9.3 cm		
Detection Scan	540 nm		
Validation Parameters	**Linearity Range:** 30-180 μg/mL **r:** 0.999 **Recovery:** 97.4%-98.6%		
Reference	58		

Stationary Phase	Silica gel GF_{254} pre-coated TLC plates		
Mobile Phase	Dichloromethane:Methanol:Water(4.5:1.0:0.1)		
Temperature	Ambient	**Compound Analyzed**	Bacoside A
Sample Volume	2 μL		
Solvent Front Migration	8 cm		
Detection Wavelength	225 nm		
Validation Parameters	**Linearity Range:** 8.4-50.4 μg/spot r^2: 0.9989 **LOD:** 3 μg **LOQ:** 9.9 μg **Recovery:** 99.46%		
Reference	59		

Stationary Phase	Silica gel 60 F_{254}, pre-coated TLC plates		
Mobile Phase	Toluene:Ethyl acetate:Formic acid:methanol (3:3:0.8:0.2)		
Temperature	25 °C	**Compound Analyzed**	Luteolin
Humidity	40%		
Sample Volume	10 μL		
Solvent Front Migration	8 cm		
Detection Scan	355 nm		
Validation Parameters	**Linearity Range:** 40-240 ng/spot r^2: 0.997 **LOD:** 25 ng **LOQ:** 40 ng **Recovery:** 100.92%		
Reference	60		

Table 2.4: Summary of HPTLC results of Bacopa monniera from selected publications

2.3.4 – Supercritical Fluid Chromatography

Agrawal and coworkers[55] reported a packed column supercritical fluid chromatographic technique with photodiode-array detection (pc-SFC-

DAD) for the separation and quantitation of bacoside A_3 and bacopaside II from Bacopa monniera. The experimental conditions were as follows:

<table>
<tr><td>Column</td><td colspan="3">Jasco Finepak Sil-5C-18 (250 x 4.6 mm, 5 μm)</td></tr>
<tr><td>Mobile Phase</td><td colspan="3">A: Supercritical CO_2
B: Methanol</td></tr>
<tr><td>Gradient</td><td colspan="3">20% to 26% B in 7.5 min</td></tr>
<tr><td>Flow Rate</td><td>2.0 mL/min</td><td rowspan="4">Compounds Analyzed</td><td rowspan="4">C1) Bacoside A_3
C2) Bacopaside II</td></tr>
<tr><td>Pressure</td><td>24 MPa</td></tr>
<tr><td>Temperature</td><td>36 °C</td></tr>
<tr><td>Detection Wavelength</td><td>210 nm</td></tr>
<tr><td rowspan="8">Validation Parameters</td><td></td><td>C1</td><td>C2</td></tr>
<tr><td>Linearity Range</td><td>10 - 120 μg/mL</td><td>10 - 150 μg/mL</td></tr>
<tr><td>r^2</td><td>0.9997</td><td>0.9992</td></tr>
<tr><td>LOD</td><td>2.5 μg/mL</td><td>4.0 μg/mL</td></tr>
<tr><td>LOQ</td><td>4.5 μg/mL</td><td>6.5 μg/mL</td></tr>
<tr><td>Recovery</td><td>99.51%</td><td>98.64%</td></tr>
<tr><td>Intra-day Variation</td><td>1.58%</td><td>1.77%</td></tr>
<tr><td>Inter-day Variation</td><td>1.86%</td><td>1.92%</td></tr>
<tr><td>Reference</td><td colspan="3">55</td></tr>
</table>

Table 2.5: SFC separation of Bacoside A3 and Bacopaside II from Bacopa monniera

2.3.5 – Enzyme-Linked Immunosorbent Assay

Enzyme-linked immunosorbent assay (ELISA) using polyclonal antibodies[61] and monoclonal antibodies[62] has been reported for the determination of pseudojujubogenin glycosides in Brahmi. It is a recommended method for screening a large number of samples with a small amount of plant materials.

References

1 A Russo, F Borrelli. Bacopa monniera, a reputed nootropic plant: an overview. Phytomedicine (2005) 12: 305-307.

2 M Rajani. "Bacopa Monnieri, a Nootropic Drug" in Bioactive Molecules and

Medicinal Plants, Edited by K G Ramawat and J M Merillon, Springer, 2008.
3 R Prasad, U S Bagde, P Puspangadan, A Varma. Bacopa monniera L.: pharmacological aspects and case study involving piriformospora indica. International Journal of Integrative Biology (2008) 3(2): 100-110.
4 Poonam Jain, Dinesh K Kulshreshtha. Bacoside A_1, a minor saponin from Bacopa monniera. Phytochemistry (1993) 33(2): 449-451.
5 Subha Rastogi, Dinesh K Kulshreshtha. Bacoside A_2, a triterpenoid saponin from Bacopa monniera. Indian Journal of Chemistry (1998) 38B: 353-356.
6 Subha Rastogi, Raghawendra Pal, Dinesh K Kulshreshtha. Bacoside A_3 – a triterpenoid saponin from Bacopa monniera. Phytochem. (1994) 36(1): 133-137.
7 R S Pawar, K K Bhutani. New dammarane triterpenoidal saponins from Bacopa monniera. Indian Journal of Chemistry (2006) 45B: 1511-1514.
8 Ajit K Chakravarty, Tapas Sarkar, Kazuo Masuda, Kenji Shiojima, Takahisa Nakane, Nobuo Kawahara. Bacopaside I and II: two pseudojujubogenin glycosides from Bacopa monniera. Phytochemistry (2001) 58: 553-556.
9 Chia-Chung Hou, Shwu-Jiuan Lin, Juei-Tang Cheng, Feng-Lin Hsu. Bacopaside III, bacopasaponin G, and bacopasides A, B and C from Bacopa monniera. J Nat. Prod. (2002) 65: 1759-1763.
10 Ajit Kumar Chakravarty, Saraswati Garai, Kazuo Masuda, Takahisa Nakane, Nobuo Kawahara. Bacopasides III–V: three new triterpenoid glycosides from Bacopa monniera. Chem. Pharm. Bull. (2003) 51(2): 215-217.
11 Yun Zhou, Yun-Heng Shen, Chuan Zhang, Juan Su, Run-Hui Liu, Wei-Dong Zhang. Triterpene saponins from Bacopa monnieri and their antidepressant effects in two mice models. J Nat prod (2007) 70: 652-655.
12 Yun Zhou, Ling Peng, Wei-Dong Zhang, De-Yun Kong. Effect of triterpenoid saponins from Bacopa monniera on scopolamine-induced memory impairment in mice. Planta medica (2009) 75(6): 568-574.
13 Chillara Sivaramakrishna, Chirravuri V Rao, Golakoti Trimurtulu, Mulabagal Vanisree, Gottumukkala V Subbaraju. Triterpenoid glycosides from Bacopa monnieri. Phytochemistry (2005) 66: 2719-2728.
14 P Bhandari, N Kumar, B Singh, I Kaur. Dammarane triterpenoid saponins from Bacopa monnieri. Can. J. Chem (2009) 87: 1230 – 1234.
15 Saraswati Garai, Shashi B Mahato, Kazuhiro Ohtani, Kazuo Yamasaki. Dammarane-type triterpenoid saponins from Bacopa monniera. Phytochemistry (1996) 42(3): 815-820.
16 Saraswati Garai, Shashi B Mahato, Kazuhiro Ohtani, Kazuo Yamasaki. Bacopasaponin D – a pseudojujubogenin glycoside from Bacopa monniera. Phytochemistry (1996) 43(2): 447-449.
17 S B Mahato, S Garai, A K Chakravarty. Bacopasaponins E and F: two jujubogenin bisdesmosides from Bacopa monniera. Phytochemistry (2000) 53: 711-714.
18 S Mandal, S Mukhopadhyay. Bacopasaponin H: a pseudojujubogenin glycoside from Bacopa monniera. Indian Journal of Chemistry (2004) 43(B): 1802-1804.
19 Ajit Kumar Chakravarty, Tapas Sarkar, Takahisa Nakane, Nobuo Kawahara, Kazuo Masuda. New phenylethanoid glycosides from Bacopa monniera.

Chem. Pharm. Bull. (2002) 50(12): 1616-1618.
20 Pamita Bhandari, Neeraj Kumar, Bikram Singh, Vijay K Kaul. Cucurbitacins from Bacopa monnieri. Phytochemistry (2007) 68: 1248-1254.
21 Rahul S Pawar, Shabana I Khan, Ikhlas A Khan. Glycosides of 20-deoxy derivatives of jujubogenin and pseudojujubogenin from Bacopa monniera. Planta Med (2007) 73: 380-383.
22 K C Bose, N K Bose. Observations on the action and uses of Herpestis monniera. Journal of the Indian Medical Association (1931) 1: 60-64.
23 R N Chopra, S L Nayar, I C Chopra. Glossary of Indian medicinal plants: Vol. 32. Council of scientific and industrial research, New Delhi, 1956.
24 M S Shastri, N S Dhalla, C L Malhotra. Chemical investigation of Herpestis monniera Linn (Brahmi). Indian J. Pharmacol. (1959) 21: 303-304.
25 Pamita Bhandari, Neeraj Kumar, Bikram Singh, Vijay Kumar Kaul. Bacosterol glycoside, a new 13,14-Seco-steroid glycoside from Bacopa monniera. Chem. Pharm. Bull. (2006) 54(2): 240-241.
26 P Bhandari, N Kumar, A P Gupta, B Singh, V K Kaul. A rapid RP – HPTLC densitometry method for simultaneous determination of major flavonoids in important medicinal plants. J. Sep. Sci (2007) 30: 2092-2096.
27 N Chatterji, R P Rastogi, M L Dhar. Chemical examination of Bacopa monniera wettst: part 1 – isolation of chemical constituents. Indian Journal of Chemistry (1963) 1(5): 212-215.
28 National Center for Biotechnology Information. PubChem Compound Database; CID=64971
http://pubchem.ncbi.nlm.nih.gov/summary/summary.cgi?cid=64971
29 National Center for Biotechnology Information. PubChem Compound Database; CID=5280794
http://pubchem.ncbi.nlm.nih.gov/summary/summary.cgi?cid=5280794
30 National Center for Biotechnology Information. PubChem Compound Database; CID=241572
http://pubchem.ncbi.nlm.nih.gov/summary/summary.cgi?cid=241572
31 National Center for Biotechnology Information. PubChem Compound Database; CID=222284
http://pubchem.ncbi.nlm.nih.gov/summary/summary.cgi?cid=222284
32 National Center for Biotechnology Information. PubChem Compound Database; CID=5281319
http://pubchem.ncbi.nlm.nih.gov/summary/summary.cgi?cid=5281319
33 National Center for Biotechnology Information. PubChem Compound Database; CID=942
http://pubchem.ncbi.nlm.nih.gov/summary/summary.cgi?cid=942
34 National Center for Biotechnology Information. PubChem Compound Database; CID=5280445
http://pubchem.ncbi.nlm.nih.gov/summary/summary.cgi?cid=5280445
35 National Center for Biotechnology Information. PubChem Compound Database; CID=5280343
http://pubchem.ncbi.nlm.nih.gov/summary/summary.cgi?cid=5280343
36 National Center for Biotechnology Information. PubChem Compound Database; CID=5280443

http://pubchem.ncbi.nlm.nih.gov/summary/summary.cgi?cid=5280443
37 National Center for Biotechnology Information. PubChem Compound Database; CID=6251 http://pubchem.ncbi.nlm.nih.gov/summary/summary.cgi?cid=6251
38 H K Singh, R P Rastogi, R C Srimal, B N Dhawan. Effect of bacosides A and B on avoidance responses in rats. Phytotherapy Research (1988) 2(2): 70-75.
39 H K Singh, B N Dhawan. Neuropsychopharmacological effects of the Ayurvedic nootropic Bacopa monniera Linn (Brahmi). Indian Journal of Pharmacology (1997) 29(5): 359-365.
40 M Deepak, A Amit. The need for establishing identities of 'bacoside A and B', the putative major bioactive saponins of Indian medicinal plant Bacopa monnieri. Phytomedicine (2004) 11: 264 – 268.
41 M Deepak, G K Sangli, P C Arun, A Amit. Quantitative determination of the major saponin mixture bacoside A in Bacopa monniera by HPLC. Phytochemical Analysis (2005) 16: 24-29.
42 A N Garg, A Kumar, A G C Nair, A V R Reddy. Elemental analysis of Brahmi (Bacopa monnieri) extracts by neutron activation and its bioassay for antioxidant, radio protective and anti-lipid peroxidation activity. J Radional Nucl Chem (2009) 281: 53-58.
43 R Pal, J P S Sarin. Quantitative determination of bacosides by UV-spectrophotometry. Indian Journal of Pharmaceutical Sciences (1992) 54: 17-18.
44 M Ganzera, J Gampenrieder, R S. Pawar, I A Khan, H Stuppener. Separation of the major triterpenoid saponins in Bacopa monnieri by high-performance liquid chromatography. Analytica Chimica Acta (2004) 516: 149-154.
45 W Phrompittayarat, S Wittaya-Areekul, K Jetiyanon, W Putalun, H Tanaka, K Ingkaninan. Determination of saponin glycosides in Bacopa monnieri by reversed phase high performance liquid chromatography. Thai Pharmaceutical and Health Science Journal (2007) 2(1): 26-32.
46 R Pal, A K Dwivedi, S Singh, D K Kulshreshtha. Quantitative determination of Bacosides by HPLC. Indian J Pharm Sci (1998) 60(5): 328-329.
47 P Bhandari, N Kumar, B Singh, V Singh, I Kaur. Silica based monolithic column with evaporative light scattering detector for HPLC analysis of bacosides and apigenin in Bacopa monnieri. J. Sep. Sci (2009) 32: 2812 – 2818.
48 P Bhandari, N Kumar, A P Gupta, B Singh, V K Kaul. Micro-LC determination of swertiamarin in Swertia species and bacoside-A in Bacopa monnieri. Chromatographia (2006) 64(9/10): 599-602.
49 P B S Murthy, V R Raju, T Ramakrisana, M S Chakravarthy, K V Kumar, S Kannababu, G V Subbaraju. Estimation of twelve Bacopa saponins in Bacopa monnieri extracts and formulations by high-performance liquid chromatography. Chem. Pharm. Bull. (2006) 54(6): 907-911.
50 T Renukappa, G Roos, I Klaiber, B Volger, W Kraus. Application of high-performance liquid chromatography coupled to nuclear magnetic resonance spectrometry, mass spectrometry and bioassay for the determination of active saponins from Bacopa monniera wettst. J. Chromatogr. A (1999) 847: 109-

116.

51 Marcello Nicoletti. Phytochemical techniques in complex botanicals. The XXI century analytical challenge. J Chromatography Separation Techniques (2012). doi: 10.4172/2157-7064.1000186

52 Joseph Sherma. Planar chromatography. Anal Chem (2008) 80: 4253-4267.

53 M Attimarad, M Ahmed K K, B E Aldhubaib, S Harsha. High performance thin layer chromatography: a powerful analytical technique in pharmaceutical drug discovery. Pharmaceutical methods (2011) 2(2): 71-75.

54 Harish Chandra Andola, Vijay Kant Purohit. High performance thin layer chromatography (HPTLC): a modern analytical tool for biological analysis. Nature and Science (2010) 8(10): 58-61.

55 H Agarwal, N Kaul, A R Paradkar, K R Mahadik. Separation of bacoside A_3 and bacopaside II, major triterpenoid saponins in Bacopa monnieri, by HPTLC and SFC. Application of SFC in implementation of uniform design for herbal drug standardization, with thermodynamic study. Acta Chromatographica (2006) 17: 125-150.

56 M D Sahare, P M D'Mello. Standardization of Bacopa monnieri and its formulations with reference to bacoside A, by high performance thin layer chromatography. International Journal of Pharmacognosy and Phytochemical Research (2010) 2(4): 8-12.

57 A P Gupta, S Mathur, M M Gupta, Sushil Kumar. Effect of the method of drying on the bacoside-A content of the harvested Bacopa monniera shoots revealed using a high performance thin layer chromatography method. Journal of Medicinal and Aromatic Plant Sciences (1998) 20: 1052-1055.

58 Sapna Shrikumar, S Sandeep, T K Ravi, M Umamaheswari. A HPTLC determination and fingerprinting of bacoside-A in Bacopa monnieri and its formulation. Indian Journal of Pharmaceutical Sciences (2004) 66(1): 132-135.

59 Om Prakash, Gyanendra N Singh, Raman M Singh, Satish C Mathur, Meenakshi Bajpai, Saroj Yadav. Determination of bacoside A by HPTLC in Bacopa monnieri extract. International Journal of Green Pharmacy (2008) 2(3): 173-175.

60 H Srinivasa, M S Bagul, H Padh, M Rajani. A rapid densitometric method for the quantification of luteolin in medicinal plants using HPTLC. Chromatographia (2004) 60(1/2): 131-134.

61 Watoo Phrompittayarat, Waraporn Putalun, Hiroyuki Tanaka, Sakchai Wittaya-Areekul, Kanchalee Jetiyanon, Kornkanok Ingkaninan. An enzyme-linked immunosorbant assay using polyclonal antibodies against bacopaside I. Analytical Chimica Acta (2007) 584: 1-6.

62 W Phrompittayarat, W Putalun, H Tanaka, K Jetiyanon, S Wittaya-Areekul, K Ingkaninan. Determination of pseudojujubogenin glycosides from Brahmi based on immunoassay using a monoclonal antibody against Bacopaside I. Phytochemical Analysis (2007) 18: 411-418.

3 – Antioxidant Activity

3.1 – General

Antioxidants protect the body from free radical damage. A free radical is a chemical entity capable of independent existence that contains one or more unpaired electrons. It may be charged or neutral. Free radicals are present almost everywhere. They are constantly produced in the body as byproducts of biochemical processes, where they can be both beneficial or harmful. When they are produced as needed, they facilitate cell survival, proliferation and differentiation[1,2]. When they are produced in an uncontrolled fashion, they can cause tissue damage and cell death. Free radicals have been implicated in the cause of several diseases and in the aging process[3].

3.2 – Reactive Oxygen and Reactive Nitrogen Species (ROS/RNS)

A free radical is represented by its chemical formula with a superscript dot to the right followed by any charge it may have. For example, $H^{\bullet}$, $HO^{\bullet}$ and $O_2^{\bullet -}$ represent hydrogen, hydroxyl and superoxide radicals, respectively. The term reactive oxygen species (ROS) refers to oxygen-containing radicals as well as some non-radical derivatives that contain oxygen. An anlogous term, reactive nitrogen species (RNS), is used for nitrogen-containing radical and non-radical derivatives.

3.3 – Formation of Free Radicals

Free radicals are generally formed by homolytic bond dissociation or single electron oxidation of an atom or molecule. Homolytic bond dissociation involves the breakup of a covalent bond in a molecule where each of the fragments carries away an electron. If atoms X and Y are covalently bonded in the molecule XY, homolytic bond dissociation between X and Y may be represented as follows:

$$X{-}Y \rightarrow X^{\bullet} + Y^{\bullet}$$

Homolytic bond dissociation in H_2 and H_2O are shown below:

$$H{-}H \rightarrow H^{\bullet} + H^{\bullet}$$

$$H{-}O{-}H \rightarrow H^{\bullet} + HO^{\bullet}$$

Oxidation is a process in which an atom or molecule loses an electron, and reduction occurs with the gain of an electron. These reactions may be represented as follows:

$$X \rightarrow X^{\bullet +} + e^{-} \quad \text{Oxidation}$$

$$Y + e^{-} \rightarrow Y^{\bullet -} \quad \text{Reduction}$$

Oxidation is always accompanied by reduction, and vice versa. Such reactions are commonly called redox reactions. The species that gives up the electron is the reducing agent (reductant) and the species that accepts the electron is the oxidizing agent (oxidant). The oxidizing power of species is estimated by their reduction potentials. The higher the reduction potential, the greater the affinity for the electron will be, and the more likely it will be reduced. The hydroxyl radical is a powerful oxidizing agent as can be inferred from its reduction potential ($E^0 = 2.31$ V for $HO^{\bullet}$, H^+/H_2O). It can react with most molecules in cells. Hydrogen peroxide has the least reactivity, highest stability, and greatest intracellular concentration of all biologically important ROS[2].

3.4 – Sources of ROS/RNS

We are constantly bombarded by free radicals from exogenous and endogenous sources. Exogenous sources include radiation, pollution, cigarette smoke, alcohol, processed food, xenobiotics, pathogens and several other sources. Although this exposure is serious, our vulnerability to endogenous sources is even greater. The human body produces numerous free radicals at various cellular locations, with mitochondria considered to be the largest source of ROS[4]. Mitochondria consume 80-90% of cellular oxygen to support oxidative phosphorylation, the metabolic pathway that harnesses energy released by the oxidation of nutrients to produce adenosine triphosphate (ATP). In this process, oxygen (O_2) undergoes a four electron reduction to water:

$$O_2 + 4\,e^{-} + 4\,H^{+} \rightarrow 2\,H_2O$$

Electrons are transferred through a chain of enzymatic complexes, I to IV. During this process, partial reduction of oxygen also occurs, and superoxide ($O_2^{\bullet -}$) is produced[5]. It is estimated that 0.1-2% of the oxygen consumed by mitochondria is partially reduced to superoxide[4-6]. Given the huge amount of oxygen consumed, even 0.1% represents a significant amount. Superoxide is converted to hydrogen peroxide (H_2O_2) by spontaneous dismutation or by superoxide dismutase (SOD). In the presence of metal ions, $HO^\bullet$ is produced via the Fenton and/or Haber-Weiss reactions[7]:

Fenton	$Fe^{2+} + H_2O_2$	$\rightarrow$	$Fe^{3+} + OH^- + HO^\bullet$

Haber-Weiss	$Fe^{3+} + O_2^{\bullet-}$	$\rightarrow$	$Fe^{2+} + O_2$
	$Fe^{2+} + H_2O_2$	$\rightarrow$	$Fe^{3+} + OH^- + HO^\bullet$
	$H_2O_2 + O_2^{\bullet-}$	$\rightarrow$	$OH^- + HO^\bullet + O_2$

In addition to mitochondria, there are other endogenous sources of ROS/RNS. The endoplasmic reticulum has a number of proteins such as cytochrome P-450, NADPH:cytochrome P-450 reductase, cytochrome b_5, NADH:cytochrome b_5 reductase, and flavin-containing monooxygenases that are involved in the metabolism of a variety of foreign compounds[8]. The microsomal mixed-function oxidase system detoxifies various compounds, but it also activates some compounds to toxic species, some of which are free radicals. Peroxisomes contain a number of enzymes that produce H_2O_2, $O_2^{\bullet-}$ and nitric oxide ($NO^\bullet$)[9]. Several enzymatic systems such as amino acid oxidases, cyclooxygenase (COX), lipoxygenase (LOX), nitric oxide synthase and xanthine oxidase in the cytosol generate $O_2^{\bullet-}$ and other derived ROS[2].

3.5 – Free Radical Reactions

Free radicals are highly reactive. Among the targets vulnerable to free radical attack are lipidic membranes, proteins, carbohydrates and DNA[10-14]. Lipidic membranes contain phospholipids, essential components of which are polyunsaturated fatty acids (PUFAs). PUFAs are highly susceptible to oxidation due to their double bonds. This type of oxidation, lipid peroxidation (LPO), is a chain reaction consisting of three steps: chain initiation, chain propagation and chain termination. In the chain initiation step, a free radical pulls off a hydrogen atom from the lipid molecule and produces a lipid radical. The lipid radical reacts with an oxygen molecule to produce a lipid peroxyl radical. The lipid peroxyl radical attacks another lipid molecule to yield lipid hydroperoxide (LHP) and another lipid radical. The process continues and the chain propagates. Chain termination occurs when a lipid radical or lipid peroxyl radical reacts with another radical or antioxidant. The three steps are shown below:

Chain Initiation	LH + X• → XH + L• *Lipid* *Lipid Radical*
Chain Propagation	L• + O_2 → LOO• *Lipid Peroxyl Radical* LOO• + LH → LOOH + L• *Lipid Hydroperoxide*
Chain Termination	LOO• + LOO• → Non radical products L• + LOO• → Non radical products L• + L• → Non radical products

Lipid peroxidation produces a variety of toxic products such as 4-hydroxy-2-nonenal (4-HNE), malondialdehyde (MDA), 2-propenal (acrolein) and isoprostane[2]. Lipid aldehydes are relatively stable, and can move out of cells and attack remote targets. Lipid peroxidation impairs membrane functions, reduces fluidity, inactivates membrane bound receptors and enzymes, and increases non-specific permeability of ions[15].

The high abundance of proteins and their reactivity make them easy targets for free radicals. Free radical attack on proteins can cause peroxidation, fragmentation, damage to amino acids, and alterations to tertiary structure[10]. Protein oxidation produces aldehydes, keto compounds and carbonyls.

DNA is a stable molecule and is well protected, but it is still susceptible to free radical attack. Free radical attack on DNA can cause strand breaks, DNA-DNA and DNA-protein cross-linking, DNA base and sugar modification, and loss of purines[10,16]. Hydroxyl radical attack on DNA produces a variety of adducts. An attack on guanine at its C-8 position produces 8-hydroxyguanosine (8-OHdG)[10]. Other positions can be attacked to produce other products. RNS attack on purines causes nitration and deamination[15]. Free radicals like HO• attack carbohydrates and abstract hydrogen atoms to produce carbon-centered radicals. This can lead to chain breaks in important molecules[17].

3.6 – Antioxidant Defense System

An antioxidant is “any substance that, when present at a low concentration relative to an oxidizable substrate, prevents or significantly delays oxidation of the substrate”[18]. To protect against free radicals, humans and other organisms have developed an intricate and efficient antioxidant defense system during the course of evolution. The first line of defense consists of preventive antioxidants. They suppress the formation of free radicals. The second line of defense consists of radical scavenging antioxidants. They remove the free radicals before they can cause damage. The third line of defense consists of enzymes that can repair damage to proteins, DNA, oxidized lipids, etc. They repair the damage, clear the waste, and restore lost functions. The body's adaptation mechanism acts as the fourth line of defense. Appropriate antioxidants are generated as and when required. Some antioxidants also act as cellular signaling messengers[19]. Both endogenous and exogenous components serve in the body's antioxidant defense system[20]. These components work synergistically to provide optimum defense against free radicals.

3.7 – Oxidative Stress and its Evaluation

Although the body is pretty well equipped to deal with free radicals, it can still be overwhelmed and suffer oxidative stress. Oxidative stress has been defined as an imbalance between oxidants and antioxidants in favor of the former[21]. While too much oxidative stress is harmful, too little oxidative stress is also unfavorable; as mentioned earlier, radicals are beneficial at certain levels. In measuring oxidative stress, direct assay of free radicals is not feasible, since they are highly reactive. Instead, the assay is usually done by measuring the end products of their reactions with biomolecules such as lipids, DNA and proteins[19]. The appearance of end products is considered evidence for the prior existence of free radicals in the cell[22]. Also, the levels of the components of the antioxidant defense system are considered to be biomarkers of oxidative stress.

3.8 – Experimental Evidence

Bacopa monniera contains a number of antioxidants such as saponins, flavonoids, phenolics and ascorbic acid. In vitro and in vivo studies have shown the antioxidant potential of Bacopa monniera.

3.8.1 – In Vitro Studies

This section describes a number of methods that have been used to assess the antioxidant capacity of Bacopa monniera.

3.8.1.1 – Diphenylpicrylhydrazyl (DPPH) Scavenging Activity

Radical scavenging assay as originally proposed by Blois[23] has been adapted to assess the free radical scavenging potential of antioxidants.

DPPH is considered a stable free radical because the lone electron is delocalized over the entire molecule[24]. An alcoholic solution of DPPH has a purple color that absorbs at 515 nm. The reduction of DPPH by an antioxidant changes the color of the solution to yellow, decreasing its absorbance at this wavelength. This change in absorbance directly correlates to the free radical scavenging capacity of the antioxidant. A variety of Bacopa monniera extracts have been evaluated with this method. The results show that most of the extracts quench DPPH, as summarized below (Table 3.1):

Extract and Standard	Results	Ref
Extract: methanol **Standard:** trolox (water soluble derivative of vitamin E)	Effect of the extract at 400 µg/mL was equivalent to 30 µM trolox.	25
Extracts: methanol (MEBM), Lipid Gelucire (50/13) (LEBM), Ayurvedic Ghrita (AGBM) **Standards:** butylated hydroxyanisole (BHA), ascorbic acid	IC_{50} (µg/mL): BHA=3.7, ascorbic acid=3.8, LEBM=5.1, MEBM=6.8, AGBM=23.1	26
Extract: methanol	IC_{50} = 0.73 mg/mL	27
Extracts: ethanol, methanol, water **Standard:** gallic acid	IC_{50} (µg/mL): gallic acid=123.56, methanol=212.08, ethanol=262.87, water=268.25	28
Extracts: methanol, water-methanol, water	Percent quenched (100 µg/mL of the extract): water-methanol ≈ 100%, water ≈ 70%, methanol < 20%	29
Extracts: hexane, petroleum ether, water, methanol **Standard:** ascorbic acid	IC_{50} (µg/mL): water=43.10, methanol=46.0, hexane=50.07, petroleum ether=52.18, ascorbic acid=78.17	30
Extracts: hexane, chloroform, ethyl acetate (EtOAc), acetone, methanol, water **Standard:** BHA	methanol was most effective and hexane least effective. IC_{50} (mg/mL): methanol=0.052, BHA=0.42	31
Extracts: ethanol, water	IC_{50} (µg/mL): water=76.42, ethanol=469	32
Extract: methanol	Dose-dependent quenching	33

Extract: ethanol **Standards**: ascorbic acid, butylated hydroxytoluene (BHT)	Percent inhibition (100 μg/mL of the extract/standard): ascorbic acid=80.38%, BHT=44.7%, ethanol=37.98%	34
Extracts: Methanol extract of Bacopa monniera (BME) and EtOAc (soluble and insoluble), n-BuOH (soluble and insoluble) and bacoside enriched (soluble and insoluble) fractions **Standard**: BHT	BME, EtOAc fraction (soluble and insoluble). n-BuOH fraction (soluble) and bacoside enriched fraction (soluble) quenched DPPH. EtOAc (soluble fraction, IC_{50} = 30 μg/mL) exhibited the highest activity. IC_{50} for BHT = 13 μg/mL	35
Extract: methanol **Standard**: ascorbic acid	IC_{50} (μg/mL): ascorbic acid=38.06, methanol=104.82	36
Extracts: water, water-methanol, ethanol. **Standard**: α–tocopherol	IC_{50} (μg/mL): α–tocopherol=29.66, water-methanol=46.40, ethanol=57.0 Water was not active.	37
Extract: methanol **Standard**: Ascorbic acid	IC_{50} (μg/mL): ascorbic acid=4.3, methanol=42.57	38
Extract: methanol **Standard**: ascorbic acid	IC_{50} (μg/mL): ascorbic acid=14.45, methanol=457.0	39
Extract: boiling water	IC_{50} = 191 μg/mL	40
Extract: ethanol **Standards**: ascorbic acid, BHA	IC_{50} (μg/mL): ascorbic acid=9.45, ethanol=79.84, BHA=14.15	41
Extract: ethanol **Standard**: BHT	IC_{50} (μg/mL): ethanol=9.41, BHT=4.16	48

Table 3.1: DPPH radical scavenging activity of Bacopa monniera

3.8.1.2 - Superoxide Scavenging Activity

As described in section 3.4, mitochondria is the most important physiological source of superoxide[5,42-44]. Besides mitochondria, there are several other sources of superoxide[44].

Superoxide is moderately reactive. It gets converted to H_2O_2 by spontaneous dismutation or by the enzyme superoxide dismutase:

$$O_2^{\bullet -} + O_2^{\bullet -} + 2\,H^+ \rightarrow O_2 + H_2O_2$$

In the presence of metal ions, highly reactive hydroxyl radicals are produced by Fenton or Haber-Weiss reactions[7]. Superoxide reacts with nitric oxide to produce the highly reactive peroxynitrite ion:

$$NO^{\bullet} + O_2^{\bullet-} \rightarrow OONO^-$$

Various extracts of Bacopa monniera have been shown to scavenge superoxide, as summarized below (Table 3.2):

Extract and Standard	Results	Ref
Extract: methanol **Standard:** SOD	25 μg/mL of extract was equivalent to 80 mU/mL of SOD	25
Extract: methanol	IC_{50} = 0.76 mg/mL	27
Extracts: hexane, petroleum ether, water, methanol **Standard:** ascorbic acid	Percent inhibition: ascorbic acid=87.8%, methanol=65.68%, water=62.34%, petroleum ether=56.67%, hexane=54.18%	30
Extract: boiling water	IC_{50} = 204 μg/mL	40
Extract: ethanol **Standard:** ascorbic acid	IC_{50} (μg/mL): ethanol=22.92, ascorbic acid=34.24	45
Extracts: hydroalcoholic, bacoside A_3 **Standards:** ascorbic acid, quercetin	IC_{50} (μg/mL): bacoside A_3=10.22, ascorbic acid=14.16, hydroalcoholic=69.33, quercetin=111.0	46
Extracts: water, hydroalcoholic **Standard:** ascorbic acid	IC_{50} (μg/mL): ascorbic acid=456.57, hydroalcoholic=495.83, water=934.06	47
Extract: ethanol **Standard:** caffeic acid	IC_{50} (μg/mL): caffeic acid=4.15, ethanol=10	48

Table 3.2: Superoxide scavenging activity of Bacopa monniera

3.8.1.3 – Hydrogen Peroxide Scavenging Activity

Hydrogen peroxide is produced by the dismutation of $O_2^{\bullet-}$ catalyzed by superoxide dismutase[10]:

$$O_2^{\bullet-} + O_2^{\bullet-} + 2\,H^+ \rightarrow O_2 + H_2O_2$$

Oxidative deamination of biogenic amines by monoamine oxidase (MAO) present in the outer membrane of mitochondria produces significant amounts of H_2O_2 [42]. Hydrogen peroxide is a non-radical ROS, and can cause damage both directly and indirectly. Its direct damage includes degradation of heme proteins, inactivation of enzymes and oxidation of DNA, lipids, -SH groups and keto acids. Indirect damage includes conversion of hydrogen peroxide to other highly reactive radicals such as $HO^{\bullet}$[10]. A number of investigations have demonstrated the hydrogen peroxide scavenging activity of Bacopa monniera and some results are presented below (Table 3.3):

Extract and Standard	Results	Ref
Extracts: methanol (MEBM), Lipid Gelucire (50/13, LEBM), Ayurvedic Ghrita (AGBM) **Standards:** BHA, ascorbic acid	IC_{50} (µg/mL): BHA=5.4, ascorbic acid=5.5, LEBM=5.58, MEBM=6.9, AEBM=14.8	26
Extract: methanol	Concentration-dependent scavenging	33
Extracts: water, hydroalcoholic **Standard:** ascorbic acid	The hydroalcoholic extract was more effective (similar to ascorbic acid).	47

Table 3.3: Hydrogen peroxide scavenging activity of Bacopa monniera

3.8.1.4 – Hydroxyl Radical Scavenging Effect

Most of the hydroxyl radicals in the body are generated through the Fenton reaction[7]. The hydroxyl radical is highly reactive, and can attack most organic and inorganic molecules in the cell including DNA, proteins, lipids, amino acids and sugars. A number of investigations have demonstrated the hydroxyl radical scavenging activity of Bacopa monniera and the results are summarized below (Table 3.4):

Extract and Standard	Results	Ref
Extracts: ethanol, methanol, water	IC_{50} (µg/mL): methanol=200, ethanol=240, water=240	28
Extracts: hexane, chloroform, EtOAc, acetone, methanol, water	IC_{50} (mg/mL): methanol=0.345, water=0.350. IC_{50} values for other extracts were between 0.45 and 0.6 mg/mL	31

Extracts: methanol extract of Bacopa monniera (BME) and EtOAc (soluble and insoluble), n-BuOH (soluble and insoluble) and bacoside enriched (soluble and insoluble) fractions **Standards:** quercetin	BME and all of the fractions except n-BuOH (insoluble) and bacoside enriched (insoluble) were active. EtOAc (soluble fraction, IC_{50} = 25 µg/mL) was the most active. IC_{50} for quercetin = 5 µg/mL	35
Extracts: water-methanol, ethanol **Standard:** mannitol	IC_{50} (µg/mL): water-methanol=41.25, ethanol=45.25, mannitol=331.31	37
Extract: boiling water	IC_{50} = 721 µg/mL	40
Extracts: water, hydroalcoholic **Standard:** ascorbic acid	IC_{50} (µg/mL): ascorbic acid=448.19, hydroalcoholic=488.0, water=510.6	47
Extract: ethanol **Standard:** BHT	IC_{50} (µg/mL): BHT=6.85, ethanol=436.77	48

Table 3.4: Hydroxyl radical scavenging activity of Bacopa monniera

3.8.1.5 – Nitric Oxide Scavenging Activity

Nitric oxide mediates a number of diverse physiological processes including vasodilatation, neurotransmission, smooth muscle relaxation and immune system regulation[44,49]. It is generated by the oxidation of the amino acid arginine catalyzed by various nitric oxide synthase enzymes[10]. During the oxidative burst triggered by the inflammation process, the immune system produces both superoxide and nitric oxide. Nitric oxide reacts with molecular oxygen, superoxide radicals, transition metal ions and other free radicals[44]. Bacopa monniera has been shown to scavenge nitric oxide by a number of investigators, and the results are summarized below (Table 3.5):

Extract and Standard	Results	Ref
Extracts: ethanol, methanol, water **Standard:** curcumin	IC_{50} (µg/mL): curcumin=150.74, methanol=285.05, water=329.49, ethanol=362.29	28
Extracts: ethanol, water	Moderate nitric oxide scavenging activity	32

Extract: methanol **Standard:** ascorbic acid	IC_{50} (µg/mL): ascorbic acid=36.16, methanol=455.78	36
Extract: methanol	IC_{50} = 337.98 µg/mL	38
Extract: methanol **Standards:** ascorbic acid, quercetin	IC_{50} (µg/mL): ascorbic acid=5.47, quercetin=15.24, methanol=21.29	39
Extract: ethanol **Standard:** ascorbic acid	IC_{50} (µg/mL): ascorbic acid=15.02, ethanol=29.17	45
Extracts: water, hydroalcoholic **Standard:** ascorbic acid	IC_{50} (µg/mL): hydroalcoholic=169.22, ascorbic acid=210.75, water=254.70	47
Extract: ethanol	IC_{50} = 9.21 µg/mL	48

Table 3.5: Nitric Oxide scavenging activity of Bacopa monniera

3.8.1.6 – Reactive Oxygen Species (ROS) Scavenging Activity

Bacopa monniera has been shown to scavenge ROS produced in many reactions. The results are summarized below (Table 3.6):

Extract and Standard	Results	Ref
Extract: water-methanol	Suppressed ROS produced in the reaction of nura-2 cells (rat neuroblast cell line) with As_2O_3	37
Extract: ethanol	Scavenged ROS produced by the incubation of mouse brain homogenate with t-butyl hydroperoxide. Incubation of homogenate with 250, 500 and 1000 µg/mL of extract reduced ROS by 71%, 78% and 81%, respectively, compared to the control.	50
Extract: methanol along with its solvent partitioned fractions: dichloromethane (DCM), EtOAc, n-BuOH, water **Standard:** trolox	All extracts inhibited ROS generation in rat kidney homogenate. IC_{50} (µg/mL): EtOAc=14.03, trolox=29.82, n-BuOH=35.29, methanol=46.52, water=65.54, DCM=98.45	51

Table 3.6: ROS scavenging activity of Bacopa monniera

3.8.1.7 - Peroxynitrite Scavenging Activity

Peroxynitrite is formed by the reaction of nitric oxide and superoxide[44]:

$$NO^{\bullet} + O_2^{\bullet -} \rightarrow OONO^-$$

$NO^{\bullet}$ and $O_2^{\bullet -}$ are also oxidants, but $OONO^-$ is more powerful. The protonated form of peroxynitrite, ONOOH, is also a powerful oxidizing agent. It can cause DNA damage, protein oxidation and nitration of aromatic amino acid residues in proteins[10].

Alam and coworkers[51] evaluated the peroxynitrite scavenging effect of Bacopa monniera. A methanol extract of Bacopa monniera and its soluble organic fractions were obtained by successive partitioning with dichloromethane (DCM), ethyl acetate (EtOAc), n-butanol (n-BuOH) and water. The methanol extract and its fractions showed $OONO^-$ scavenging activity. The effect decreased in the order EtOAc (IC_{50}=1.03 μg/mL) > n-BuOH (IC_{50}=3.29 μg/mL) > methanol (IC_{50}=11.23 μg/mL) > water (IC_{50}=25.54 μg/mL) > DCM (IC_{50}=55.52 μg/mL). The IC_{50} value for penicillamine (standard) was 1.17 μg/mL.

3.8.1.8 - Reducing Power

A number of investigators have determined the reducing power of different extracts of Bacopa monniera and the results are summarized below (Table 3.7):

Extract and Standard	Reducing Power	Ref
Extracts: methanol (MEBM) Lipid Gelucire (50/13, LEBM), Ayurvedic Ghrita of Brahmi (AGBM)	IC_{50} (μg/mL): LEBM=415.75, MEBM=718.2, AGBM=736.4	26
Extract: methanol	concentration-dependent	27
Extracts: ethanol, methanol, water	ethanol > methanol > water	28
Extracts: hexane, chloroform, ethyl acetate, acetone, methanol, water	methanol > water > acetone > ethyl acetate chloroform and hexane did not show reducing capacity	31
Extracts: ethanol, water	concentration-dependent	32
Extract: methanol **Standard:** BHT	Similar to BHT	33
Extract: ethanol **Standards:** BHT, ascorbic acid	Less reducing power than BHT or ascorbic acid	34

Extract: methanol **Standards:** ascorbic acid, gallic acid	Similar to ascorbic acid. IC_{50} (µg/mL): gallic acid=58.26, methanol=96.1	36
Extracts: water, water-methanol, ethanol **Standards:** ascorbic acid, gallic acid	gallic acid > ascorbic acid > ethanol > water-methanol > water	37
Extract: methanol	Showed reducing power	38
Extract: methanol **Standard:** ascorbic acid	Similar to ascorbic acid	39
Extract: ethanol **Standard:** ascorbic acid	Similar to ascorbic acid	45
Extract: water, hydroalcoholic	hydroalcoholic > water	47

Table 3.7: Reducing power of Bacopa monniera

3.8.1.9 – Effect of Bacopa monniera on divalent iron chelation

Dhanasekaran and coworkers[50] demonstrated the iron-chelating property of Bacopa monniera. Removal of Fe^{2+} by chelation makes it unavailable for the Fenton reaction. An ethanol extract (25-100 µg) of Bacopa monniera was added to ferrozine and the reaction was monitored at 562 nm. The extract decreased the concentration of Fe^{2+} in a dose-dependent manner. Shinomol and coworkers[48] also showed a concentration-dependent iron chelation effect of an ethanol extract (IC_{50}=160 µg/mL). IC_{50} for EDTA was 50 µg/mL.

3.8.1.10 – Anti-Lipid Peroxidation Activity

A number of investigators have evaluated the effect of Bacopa monniera on lipid peroxidation.

Tripathy and coworkers[52] found that alcoholic and hexane extracts of Bacopa monniera inhibited LPO induced by ferrous sulfate or cumene hydroperoxide in rat liver homogenate. The alcohol extract was more effective than the hexane extract. ED_{50} values for the alcohol extract were 100 µg and 177 µg in reactions induced by ferrous sulfate and cumene hydroperoxide, respectively. For the hexane extract, the corresponding ED_{50} values were 290 µg and 400 µg. The effect of the alcohol extract on LPO induced by ferrous sulfate was compared to the effects of 2-amino-2(hydroxymethyl)-1,3-propanediol (tris, a hydroxyl trapper), ethylenediaminetetraacetic acid (EDTA, a divalent metal ion chelator) and Vitamin E (a natural chain breaking antioxidant). EDTA, Vitamin E and the alcohol extract of Bacopa monniera showed a dose-dependent inhibitory effect, whereas tris showed no effect. ED_{50} values for Vitamin E, the alcohol extract and EDTA were 58 μg, 100 μg and 247 μg, respectively.

It was also observed that the Bacopa extract exerted very little effect on the aerial or ferrous sulfate induced oxidation of glutathione in liver homogenate. It was suggested that Bacopa monniera might function as a metal chelator at the initial level and also as a chain-breaker, but not as a regulator of glutathione.

Results from several other studies are presented below (Table 3.8):

Extract and Standard	Results	Ref
Extracts: methanol (MEBM), Lipid Gelucire (LEBM), Ayurvedic Ghrita of Brahmi (AGBM) **Standards:** BHA, ascorbic acid	Inhibited LPO in rat liver homogenate induced by ferric chloride. IC_{50} (μg/mL): BHA=4.02, LEBM=4.4, MEBM=4.7, ascorbic acid=4.10, AGBM=5.7	26
Extract: methanol	Inhibited $FeSO_4$/ascorbic acid induced LPO in rat liver microsomes (IC_{50} = 0.72 mg/mL)	27
Extracts: methanol, water-methanol and water	Showed dose-dependent inhibition of LPO induced by Fe^{2+}/ascorbate and AAPH protocols. The water-methanol extract was more potent than the other two in both the Fe^{2+}/ascorbate (IC_{50} = 8.57 μg/mL) and AAPH (IC_{50} = 144 μg/mL) systems	29
Extracts: ethanol, water	Inhibited LPO induced by $FeCl_3$ in the goat brain, ethanol > water	32
Extract: water-methanol **Standard:** BHT	Inhibited LPO induced by $FeSO_4$ /ascorbate in rat brain mitochondria. ethanol (100 μg/mL) was similar to BHT (0.2 mM)	37
Extract: boiling water	Inhibited $FeSO_4$ induced LPO in egg yolk homogenate. IC_{50} = 345 μg/mL	40
Extract: ethanol **Standard:** α-tocopherol	Inhibited $FeCl_2$-ascorbic acid induced LPO in rat liver tissues. IC_{50} (μg/mL): α-tocopherol=133.86, ethanol=154.51	45

Extracts: water, hydroalcoholic **Standard:** ascorbic acid	Inhibited LPO induced by Fe^{2+}/ascorbate in rat liver homogenate, hydroalcoholic > water. The hydroalcoholic extract was comparable to ascorbic acid.	47
Extract: ethanol	Inhibited hydrogen peroxide induced LPO in mouse brain homogenate.	50

Table 3.8: Anti-lipid peroxidation activity of Bacopa monniera

3.8.1.11 – Phenolic, Flavonoid and Anthocyanin Content

Polyphenols, flavonoids and anthocyanins occur abundantly in a number of plants and are known for their antioxidant activity. Various extracts of Bacopa monniera have been shown to contain significant amounts of these compounds. Some results are summarized below (Table 3.9):

Extract	Results	Ref
Methanol (MEBM), Lipid Gellucire (50/13, LEBM), Ayurvedic Ghrita (AGBM)	Phenolic and flavonoid content: LEBM > MEBM > AGBM	26
Ethanol, methanol, water	Showed phenolic and flavonoid content	28
Methanol, water-methanol, water	Showed considerable phenolic content	29
Hexane, petroleum ether, water, methanol	Phenolic content (μg of gallic acid equivalents (GAE)/g of the plant material): hexane=59.1, petroleum ether=88.0, water=107.5, methanol=241.3	30
Hexane, chloroform, EtOAc, acetone and water	Polyphenol content: methanol > water > chloroform > acetone > EtOAc > hexane. GAE (μg/mL): methanol=55, water=52	31
Ethanol, water	Phenolic content (μg/mL of GAE): water=3.71, ethanol=3.18 Flavonoid content (μg/mL of quercetin equivalents (QE)): ethanol=115, water=85.63	32
Methanol	Total phenols estimate: 0.83% catechol quivalent (CE)	33

Water (BA), water-methanol (BAM), ethanol (BE)	Phenolic content (µg of GAE/mg of plant extract): BE=87.75, BAM=82.25, BA=29.25 Flavonoid content (epicatechin equivalent/mg of plant extract): BAM=95.90, BE=81.45, BA=36.25	37
Methanol	Polyphenols = 63.2 mg GAE/g extract Flavonoids = 60 mg CE/g extract Anthocyanins = 0.5 µmol/g extact	38
Methanol	Phenolic content = 21.54 mg/g GAE Flavonoid content = 24.36 mg/g QE	39
Boiling water	Phenol content = 118 ug GAE/mg of plant material	40
Ethanol	Phenolic content was 47.7 µg of pyrocatechol/mg extract	45
Water, hydroalcoholic	Phenolic content (mg GAE/g of extract): hydroalcoholic=116.1, water=58 Flavonoid content (mg CE/g of extract): hydroalcoholic=242.6, water=202.8	47
Ethanol	Polyphenol content = 51.8 µg/mg	50

Table 3.9: Phenolic, flavonoid, flavonol and anthocyanin content of Bacopa monniera

3.8.2 – In Vivo Studies

The antioxidant activity of Bacopa monniera in rodents has been determined by inducing oxidative changes through various methods. Results from some published studies are summarized below.

Bhattacharya and coworkers[53] showed the antioxidant activity of a Bacopa monniera extract (BM) in various parts of the rat brain. Adult male Wistar rats treated with BM (5 or 10 mg/kg/day, PO) for 14 or 21 days showed dose-dependent increases in SOD, CAT and GPx in the frontal cortex, striatum and hippocampus compared to the control group. The effect was more pronounced after 21 days. Rats treated with the neurological antioxidant L-deprenyl (2 mg/kg/day, PO) showed increased SOD, CAT and GPx in the frontal cortex and striatum, but not in the hippocampus.

Gajare and coworkers[54] examined the effect of an alcoholic extract of Bacopa monniera (BM) on oxidative damage induced by D-galactose in the mouse brain. Female albino mice treated with D-galactose (5%, 0.5

mL/day, SC) for 15 days showed increased LPO and decreased SOD, CAT and GPx compared to the control group. Mice treated with D-galactose (5%) containing BM (40 mg/kg/day, SC) showed a reversal of these changes.

Jyothi and Sharma[55] evaluated the effect of an alcoholic extract of Bacopa monniera (BME) on oxidative stress induced by aluminum chloride in the rat hippocampus. Male Wistar rats treated with $AlCl_3$ in drinking water (50 mg/kg/day, PO) for 5 weeks showed increased LPO and protein oxidation, and decreased SOD activity in the hippocampus compared to the control group. Rats treated with $AlCl_3$ in drinking water (50 mg/kg/day, PO) and either BM (40 mg/kg/day, PO) or L-deprenyl (1 mg/kg/day) intraperitoneally (i.p.) for 5 weeks showed a reversal of these changes. The effect of BME was similar to L-deprenyl. The authors concluded that **"Bacopa's neuroprotective effects were comparable to those of L-deprenyl at both biochemical and microscopic levels."**

In a subsequent investigation, Jyothi and coworkers[56] showed that an ethanol extract of Bacopa monniera decreased aluminum-induced oxidative stress in the cerebral cortex of rat brains. Rats treated with $AlCl_3$ (50 mg/kg/day, PO) for 5 weeks showed an increase in LPO and protein oxidation, and a decrease in SOD, glutathione-S-transferase (GST), GPx and glutathione (GSH) in the cerebral cortex compared to the control group. Also, the accumulation of lipofuscin pigment and chromatin condensation was greater in the $AlCl_3$ treated rats compared to the control group. Coadministration of Bacopa monniera extract (40 mg/kg/day, PO) or L-deprenyl (1 mg/kg/day, i.p.) reduced the $AlCl_3$ induced changes. The authors concluded that **"these findings strongly implicate that Bacopa monniera has potential to protect brain from oxidative damage resulting from aluminum toxicity."**

Madhavi and coworkers[57] reported that treatment of male albino rats (3 months old) with aluminum maltolate (100 mg/kg/day, PO) for 1 month increased LPO and decreased SOD, CAT and GPx in the medulla oblongata compared to the control group. Rats treated with aluminum maltolate and an alcoholic extract of Bacopa monniera (40 mg/kg/day, PO) for 1 month showed a reversal of these changes.

Tripathy and coworkers[58] showed that treatment of aged rats (24 months old) with $AlCl_3$ (100 mg/kg/day) for 90 days increased ROS, protein carbonyl (PC), lipofuscin (LIF), LPO, oxidized glutathione (GSSG) and acetylcholinesterase (AChE) activity, and decreased SOD, CAT, GPx, glutathione reductase (GR) and GSH in the cerebellum compared to the control group. Rats treated with $AlCl_3$ and either an ethanol extract of Bacopa monniera (40 mg/kg/day) or donepezil (2.5 mg/kg/day) for 90 days showed a reversal of these changes. The authors concluded that **"B monnieri may prove efficacious in ameliorating the aluminum induced alterations in neuromuscular and cognitive behavior and neurochemical changes in aged rat cerebellum."**

Vijayan and Helen[59] showed that a cold water extract of Bacopa monniera (BAE) mitigated the oxidative stress induced by nicotine in the mouse liver. Male albino Swiss mice treated with Nicotine (0.6 mg/kg/day, i.p.) for 7 days showed increased LPO and decreased SOD, CAT, GPx and GSH in the liver compared to the control group. Mice treated with Nicotine and BAE (50 mg/kg/day, i.p.) for 7 days showed a reversal of these changes.

Anbarsi and coworkers[60] found that bacoside A protected the rat brain from oxidative damage caused by chronic exposure to cigarette smoke. Adult male albino Wistar rats exposed to cigarette smoke twice daily (3 hrs per exposure) for 12 weeks showed the following changes compared to the control group:

- Decreased SOD, CAT, GPx and GR (brain)
- Decreased serum ceruloplasmin activity
- Decreased Zn and Se and increased Cu and Fe (brain)
- Decreased GSH, Vitamin C, Vitamin E and Vitamin A (brain)

Rats exposed to cigarette smoke and treated with bacoside A (10 mg/kg/day, PO) for 12 weeks showed a reversal of these changes. The authors concluded that **"Bacoside A ameliorates cigarette smoke induced oxidative changes probably through its free radical scavenging, antilipid peroxidative and antioxidant activities in the brain tissue."**

Palaniswamy and coworkers[61] showed that a methanol extract of Bacopa monniera leaves (BM) mitigated the oxidative stress induced by alcohol and alcohol + carbon tetrachloride in the rat liver and kidney. Male Wistar albino rats treated with alcohol (10%, 20 days) in drinking water or with alcohol (10%, 20 days) + CCl_4 (2.0 mL/kg, SC, day 21) showed decreased SOD, CAT and peroxidase in the liver and kidney compared to the control group. The effect of alcohol + CCl_4 was greater than the effect of alcohol alone. Rats treated with BM (500 mg/kg/day, 21 days) or silymarin (25 mg/kg/day, 21 days) showed a reversal of the changes induced by alcohol or alcohol + CCl_4. Silymarin (a standard hepatoprotective antioxidant) was more effective than BM. The authors concluded that **"Bacopa monniera can be used as a potential antioxidant and hepatoprotective agent."**

Sumathi and coworkers[62] demonstrated the antioxidant effect of an alcohol extract of Bacopa monniera (BME) against methyl mercury (MeHg) induced oxidative stress in the cerebellum of rats. Methyl mercury, a neurotoxin, is a ubiquitous environmental pollutant. Male albino rats treated with MeHg (5 mg/kg/day, PO) for 21 days showed the following changes compared to the control group:

- Deficit in motor performance
- Increased LPO, PC and GR (cerebellum)
- Decreased SOD, CAT and GPx activity (cerebellum)

Rats treated with MeHg and BME (40 mg/kg/day, PO) for 21 days showed a reversal of these changes. The investigators concluded that "**Bacopa monniera extract might be a potential candidate for reducing MeHg induced oxidative stress in rats.**"

Verma and coworkers[63] reported the effectiveness of an ethanol extract of Bacopa monniera (BM) in preventing oxidative changes induced by decabromodiphenyl ether (PBDE-209) in the frontal cortex (FC) and hippocampus (HC) of neonate and young mice. Male Swiss albino mice pups from the same litter treated with PBDE-209 (20 mg/kg/day, PO) from postnatal day (PND) 3 to 10 showed the following changes compared to the control group:

- Impairment of spatial memory and learning
- Increased LPO and PC (FC and HC)
- Decreased SOD and GPx (FC and HC)

Mice treated with PBDE-209 and BM (120 mg/kg/day, PO) from PND-3 to PND-10 showed a reversal of these changes.

Shobhana and Sumati[64] showed that bacoside A attenuated oxidative changes induced by 6-hydroxydopamine (6-OHDA) in the rat brain. Male albino rats (5 months old) were treated with the vehicle (ascorbic acid-saline) intracranially for 21 days. On day 22, 6-OHDA in ascorbic acid-saline was injected into the right striatum. These rats showed increased LPO and decreased GSH in the substantia nigra and decreased GST, GPx, GR, SOD and CAT in the striatum compared to the control group. Rats treated with bacoside A (10 or 20 mg/kg/day, PO) for 21 days and lesioned with 6-OHDA on day 22 showed a reversal of these changes.

Shinomol and coworkers[65] investigated the effect of an alcohol extract of Bacopa monniera on rotenone-induced oxidative stress in the prepubertal mouse brain. Rotenone is a pesticide that has been reported to cause motor impairment and behavior deficits, oxidative stress and neurodegeneration. Prepubertal male mice (4 week-old Swiss) treated with rotenone (1 mg/kg/day, i.p.) for 7 days showed the following changes in the cytosolic fractions prepared from various brain regions compared to the control group:

- Increased LPO, PC, ROS and hydroperoxide (HP)
- Decreased GSH, CAT, GPx and GR
- Increased GST, SOD, AChE and BuChE
- Decreased dopamine (striatum)

Mice treated with rotenone and BME (5 mg/kg/ day, i.p.) for 7 days showed a reversal of these changes. The authors concluded that "**Collectively our findings provide reasonable evidence on the neuroprotective effect of BME in several brain regions, which is suggestive of the broad neuro-therapeutic potential of the Ayurvedic herb in mitigating oxidative stress-mediated neuronal dysfunction.**"

Shinomol and Muralidhara[66] investigated the antioxidant effect of Bacopa monniera (leaf powder) in the prepubertal mouse brain. Prepubertal male mice (4 weeks old) treated with a powdered commercial diet fortified with Bacopa monniera leaf powder (0.5% or 1%) for 4 weeks showed the following changes in the cytosolic and mitochondrial preparations obtained from various brain regions compared to the control group:

- Decreased LPO, ROS and protein oxidation
- Increased GSH and thiol levels
- Increased CAT, GPx and SOD
- Decreased AChE activity

The authors stated that "**it is hypothesized that dietary intake of BM leaf powder confers neuroprotective advantage and is likely to be effective as a prophylactic/therapeutic agent for neurodegenerative disorders involving oxidative stress.**"

In a subsequent investigation, Shinomol and coworkers[48] demonstrated the prophylactic efficacy of an alcohol extract of Bacopa monniera (leaf) against 3-NPA induced oxidative stress in the mouse brain. Prepubertal mice treated with saline for 10 days and challenged with 3-NPA (75 mg/kg, i.p.) on days 9 and 10 showed the following changes in the cytosolic preparations from various brain regions compared to the control group:

- Increased LPO, PC, ROS and HP
- Decreased GSH, thiols, CAT, GPx and SOD

Mice treated with the Bacopa monniera extract (5 mg/kg/day, PO) for 10 days and challenged with 3-NPA on days 9 and 10 showed a reversal of these changes. The authors stated that **"it is hypothesized that BME can serve as a useful adjuvant in protecting brain against oxidative-mediated neurodegenerative disorders involving oxidative stress conditions."**

Also, Shinomol and coworkers[67] showed that pretreatment with Bacopa monniera extract mitigated 3-NPA induced mitochondrial oxidative stress and dysfunctions in the striatum of the prepubertal mouse brain.

Priyanka and coworkers[68] showed that treatment of female Wistar rats (3 months old) with Bacopa monniera for 10 days modulated the activities of antioxidant enzymes in the brain, heart and lymphoid organs. The observations of rats treated with Bacopa monniera compared to the control group are summarized below:

- Increased SOD activity in the thymus and mesenteric lymph nodes and decreased SOD activity in the medial basal hypothalamus and hippocampus
- Increased CAT activity in the spleen, frontal cortex, striatum and hippocampus
- Increased GPx activity in the heart, thymus, spleen, medial basal hypothalamus, striatum and hippocampus

Priyanka and coworkers[69] investigated the antioxidant effect of Bacopa monniera in lymphocytes isolated from the spleen of rats belonging to different age groups. Young (3-month old), early middle aged (8-9 month old) and old (18 month old) male F344 rats were sacrificed, and the splenic lymphocytes were isolated. Lymphocytes were incubated with Concanavalin A (Con A) and various concentrations of Bacopa monniera. Lymphocytes not treated with Bacopa monniera served as the control. The observations from this study are summarized below:

- Old rats showed less SOD activity compared to young and early middle-aged rats. Young rats treated with Bacopa monniera showed decreased SOD activity compared to the corresponding control group.
- There was an age-dependent decrease in the activities of CAT, GPx and GST in untreated rats: young > early middle-aged > old. Young and early middle-aged rats treated with Bacopa monniera showed increased CAT, GPx and GST activity compared to the corresponding control group. Old rats treated with Bacopa monniera showed increased GPx and GST activity compared to the corresponding control group.
- There was an age-dependent increase in LPO: young < early middle-aged < old. Young, middle-aged and old rats treated with

Bacopa monniera showed decreased LPO compared to the corresponding control group.

References

1 Andreas M Papas. "Determinants of antioxidant status in humans" in Antioxidant Status, Diet, Nutrition and Health. Edited by Andreas M Papas. CRC press, Boca Raton, FL, 1998.
2 M Mari, A Colell, A Morales, C von Montfort, C Garcia-Ruiz, J C Fernandez-Checa. Redox control of liver function in health and disease. Antioxidants and Redox Signaling (2010) 12(11): 1295-1331.
3 Barry Halliwell, John M C Gutteridge. Free Radicals in Biology and Medicine. Clarendon Press, Oxford, UK, 1999.
4 Giuseppe Paradies, Giuseppe Petrosillo, Valeria Paradies, Francesca M Ruggiero. Oxidative Stress, mitochondrial bioenergetics and cardiolipin in aging. Free Radical Biology & Medicine (2010) 48: 1286-1295.
5 David Hernandez-Garcia, Christopher D Wood, Susana Castro-Obregon, Luis Covarrubias. Reactive oxygen species: a radical role in development? Free Radical Biology & Medicine (2010) 49: 130-143.
6 Magdalena L Circu, Tak Yew Aw. Reactive oxygen species, cellular redox systems and apoptosis. Free Radical Biology & Medicine (2010) 48: 749-762.
7 V Niviere, M Fontecave. "Biological sources of reduced oxygen species" in Analysis of Free Radicals in Biological Systems. Edited by A E Favier, J Cadet, B Kalyanaraman, M Fontecave, J L Pierre. Birkhauser, Basel 1995.
8 Charles R Myers. "Subcelluar sites of xenobiotic-induced free-radical generation" in Free Radical Toxicology. Edited by Kendall B Wallace. Taylor and Francis, Washington, 1997.
9 Oksana Ivashchenko, Paul P Van Veldhoven, Chantal Brees, Ye-Shih Ho, Stanley R. Terlecky, Marc Fransen. Intraperoxisomal redox balance in mammalian cells: oxidative stress and interorganellar cross-talk. Molecular Biology of the Cell (2011) 22: 1440-1451.
10 Ron Kohen, Abraham Nyska. Oxidation of biological systems: oxidative stress phenomena, antioxidants, redox reactions and methods for Their quantification. Toxicologic Pathology (2002) 30(6): 620-650.
11 Noriko Noguchi, Etsuo Niki. "Chemistry of active oxygen species and antioxidants" in Antioxidant Status, Diet, Nutrition and Health. Edited by Andreas M Papas. CRC Press, Boca Raton, FL, 1998.
12 Kelvin J A Davies. Protein damage and degradation by oxygen radicals. The Journal of Biological Chemistry (1987) 262(20): 9895-9901.
13 Kenneth B Beckman, Bruce N Ames. Oxidative decay of DNA. The Journal of Biological Chemistry (1997) 272(32): 19633-19636.
14 R L Levine, E R Stadtman. Oxidative modifications of proteins during aging. Exp Gerontology (2001) 36(9): 1495-1502.
15 B Palmieri, V Sblendorio. Oxidative stress tests: overview on reliability and use part 1. European Review for Medical and Pharmacological Sciences (2007) 11: 309-342.
16 W R Markesbery, M A Lovell. Damage to lipids, proteins, DNA, and RNA

in mild cognitive impairment. Archives of Neurology (2007) 64(7): 954-956.

17 T P A Devasagayam, J C Tilak, K K Boloor, Ketaki S Sane, Saroj S Ghaskadbi, R D Lele. Free radicals and antioxidants in human health: current status and future prospects. JAPI (2004) 52: 794-804.

18 Barry Halliwell. "Free radicals and other reactive species in disease" in Encyclopedia of Life Sciences. John Wiley & Sons Ltd, Chichester, 2005. doi: 10.1038/npg.els.0003913

19 Etsuo Niki. Assessment of antioxidant capacity in vitro and in vivo. Free Radical Biology & Medicine (2010) 49: 503-515.

20 Robert A Jacob. The integrated antioxidant system. Nutrition Research (1995) 15(5): 755-766.

21 Helmut Sies. "Oxidative stress: introductory remarks" in Oxidative Stress. Edited by Helmut Sies. Academic Press, London, 1985.

22 Garry J Handelman, William A Pryor. "Evaluation of antioxidant status in humans" in Antioxidant Status, Diet, Nutrition and Health. Ed. Andreas M. Papas, CRC Press, Boca Raton, FL, 1998.

23 Marsden S Blois. Antioxidant determinations by the use of a stable free radical. Nature (1958) 181: 1199-1200.

24 Phillip Molyneux. The use of stable free radical diphenylpicryl-hydrazyl (DPPH) for estimating antioxidant activity. Songklanakarin J. Sci. Technol. (2004) 26(2): 211-219.

25 Alessandra Russo, Angelo A Izzo, Francesca Borrelli, Marcella Renis, Angelo Vanella. Free radical scavenging capacity and protective effect of Bacopa monniera L. on DNA damage. Phytotherapy Research (2003) 17: 870-875.

26 Lohidasan Sathiyanarayanan, Anant R Paradkar, Kakasaheb R Mahadik. In vivo and in vitro antioxidant activity of lipid based extract of Bacopa monniera Linn. compared to conventional extract and traditional preparation. European Journal of Integrative Medicine (2010) 2: 93-101.

27 A D Sathisha, H B Lingaraju, K Sham Prasad. Evaluation of antioxidant activity of medicinal plant extracts produced for commercial Purpose. E-Journal of Chemistry (2011) 8(2): 882-886.

28 M Manjula, S Anitha, S Shashidhara. Comparative evaluation of antioxidant potential and total phenolic content in selected medicinal plants. Journal of Pharmacy Research (2011) 4(4): 1065-1066.

29 A N Garg, A Kumar, A G C Nair, A V R Reddy. Elemental analysis of Brahmi (Bacopa monnieri) extracts by neutron activation and its bioassay for antioxidant, radio protective and anti-lipid peroxidation activity. J. Radioanal Nucl Chem (2009) 281: 53-58.

30 Dua Virender Kumar, Mathur Abishek, Verma Satish Kumar, Singh Santosh Kumar, Prasad GBKS. Phytochemical investigation and in vitro antioxidant activity of some medicinally important plants of Uttarakhand. International Research Journal of Pharmacy (2011) 2(6): 116-122.

31 Anand T, Mahadeva Naika, Swamy MSL, Farhath Khanum. Antioxidant and DNA damage preventive properties of Bacopa monniera (L) wettst. Free Rad. Antiox. (2011) 1(1): 84-90.

32 Sourav Mukherjee, Swapnil Dugad, Rahul Bhandare, Nayana Pawar, Suresh Jagtap, Pankaj K Pawar, Omkar Kulkarni. Evaluation of comparative free-

radical quenching potential of Brahmi (Bacopa monnieri) and mandookaparni (Centella asiatica). AYU (2011) 32(2): 258-264.
33 Harsahay Meena, Hemant Kumar Pandey, Pankaj Pandey, Mahesh Chand Arya, Zakwan Ahmed. Evaluation of antioxidant activity of two important memory enhancing medicinal plants Bacopa monnieri and Centella asiatica. Indian J Pharmacology (2012) 44(1): 114-117.
34 P Padmanabhan, S N Jangle. Evaluation of DPPH radical scavenging activity and reducing power of four selected medicinal plants and their combinations. IJPSDR (2012) 4(2): 143-146.
35 V Viji, A Helen. Inhibition of lipoxygenases and cyclooxygenase-2-enzymes by extracts isolated from Bacopa monniera (L.) wettst. Journal of Ethnopharmacology (2008) 118: 305-311.
36 Sharan Suresh Volluri, Srinivasa Rao Bammidi, Seema Chaitanya Chippada, Meena Vangalapati. In-vitro antioxidant activity and estimation of total phenolic content in methanolic extract of Bacopa monniera. RJC (2011) 4(2): 381-386.
37 Sandip K Bandyopadhyay. Ischaemia induced oxidative stress in brain and its management with natural anti-oxidants. Bombay Hospital Journal (2009) 51(4): 460-471.
38 M H Basar, S J Hossain, S K Sadhu, M H Rahman. A comparative study of antioxidant potential of commonly used antidiabetic plants in Bangladesh. Orient Pharm Exp Med (2013) 13(1): 21-28.
39 Nur Alam, Tania Binte Wahed, Farhana Sultana, Jamiuddin Ahmed, Moynul Hasan. In vitro antioxidant potential of the methanolic extract of Bacopa monnieri L. Turk J Pharm Sci (2012) 9(3): 285-292.
40 Nabasree Dasgupta, Bratati De. Antioxidant activity of some leafy vegetables of India: a comparative study. Food Chemistry (2007) 101(2): 471-474.
41 S K Biswas, J Das, A Chowdhury, U K Karmarkar, H Hossain. Evaluation of antinociceptive and antioxidant activities of whole plant extract of Bacopa monniera. Research Journal of Medicinal Plant (2012) 6(8) 607-614.
42 E Cadenas, K J A Davies. Mitochondrial free radical generation, oxidative stress and aging. Free Radical Biology & Medicine (2000) 29(3/4): 222-230.
43 Alicia J Kowaltowski, Nadja C de Souza-Pinto, Roger F Castilho, Anibal E Vercesi. Mitochondria and reactive oxygen species. Free Radical Biology & Medicine (2009) 47: 333-343.
44 M Valko, C J Rhodes, J Moncol, M Izakovic, M Mazur. Free radicals, metals and antioxidants in oxidative stress-induced cancer. Chemico-Biological Interactions (2006) 160: 1-40.
45 Tirtha Ghosh, Tapan Kumar Maity, Mrinmay Das, Anindya Bose, Deepak Kumar Dash. In vitro antioxidant and hepatoprotective activity of ethanolic extract of Bacopa monnieri Linn. aerial parts. IJPT (2007) 6(1): 77-85.
46 Rahul Pawar, Chitra Gopalakrishnan, K K Bhutani. Dammarane triterpene saponin from Bacopa monniera as the superoxide inhibitor in polymorphonuclear cells. Planta Med (2001) 67: 752-754.
47 Chandakamadhu, S Arunkumar, P Somasekharreddy, G Prithviraj, P Johnathan, J Swapna, A Sambasivarao. Phytochemical screening and in vitro antioxidant activity of aqueous and hydroalcoholic extract of Bacopa

monnieri Linn. Pharmanest (2012) 3(5): 243-256.
48 G K Shinomol, MM S Bharath, Muralidhara. Neuromodulatory propensity of Bacopa monnieri leaf extract against 3-nitropropionic acid-induced oxidative stress: in vitro and in vivo evidences. Neurotox Res (2012) 22: 102-114.
49 Cleva Villanueva, Cecilia Giulivi. Subcellular and cellular locations of nitric oxide synthase isoforms as determinants of health and disease. Free Radical Biology & Medicine (2010) 49: 307-316.
50 Muralikrishnan Dhanasekaran, Binu Tharakan, Leigh A Holcomb, Angie R Hitt, Keith A Young, Bala V Manyam. Neuroprotective mechanisms of Ayurvedic antidementia botanical Bacopa monniera. Phytotherapy Research (2007) 21: 965-969.
51 M B Alam, M S Hossain, M Assadujjaman, M M Islam, M E H Mazumder, M E Haque. Peroxynitrite scavenging and toxicity potential of different fractions of the aerial parts of Bacopa monniera linn. IJSPR (2010) 1(10): 78-83.
52 Yamini B Tripathi, Savita Chaurasia, Ekta Tripathi, Anil Upadhyay, G P Dubey. Bacopa monniera Linn. as an antioxidant: mechanism of action. Indian Journal of Experimental Biology (1996) 34: 523-526.
53 S K Bhattacharya, A Bhattacharya, A Kumar, S Ghosal. Antioxidant activity of Bacopa monniera in rat frontal cortex, striatum and hippocampus. Phytotherapy Research (2000) 14: 174-179.
54 K A Gajare, A A Deshmukh, M M Pillai. Protective effect of Bacopa monniera on the brain of D-galactose induced aging in female albino mice. Indian Journal of Gerontology (2006) 20(3): 181-192.
55 Amar Jyoti, Deepak Sharma. Neuroprotective role of Bacopa monniera extract against aluminum-induced oxidative stress in the hippocampus of rat brain. NeuroToxicology (2006) 27: 451-457.
56 Amar Jyoti, Pallavi Sethi, Deepak Sharma. Bacopa monniera prevents from aluminum neurotoxicity in the cerebral cortex of rat brain. Journal of Ethnopharmacology (2007) 111: 56-62.
57 T Madhavi, B Mahitha, K Mallikarjuna, N John Sushma. Therapeutic effect of Bacopa monniera against aluminum induced toxicity in medulla oblongata of albino rat. J. Med. Sci. (2013) 13(6): 465-470.
58 S Tripathi, A A Mahdi, M Hasan, K Mitra, F Mahdi. Protective potential of Bacopa monniera (Brahmi) extract on aluminum induced cerebellar toxicity and associated neuromuscular status in aged rats. Cell. Mol. Biol. (2011) 57(1): 3-15.
59 Viji Vijayan, A Helen. Protective activity of Bacopa monniera Linn. on nicotine-induced toxicity in mice. Phytotherapy Research (2007) 21: 378-381.
60 K Anbarasi, G Vani, K Balakrishna, C S Shyamala Devi. Effect of bacoside A on brain antioxidant status in cigarette smoke exposed rats. Life Sciences (2006) 78: 1378-1384.
61 Radha Palaniswamy, Sumathi Sundaravadivelu, Padma Palghat Raghunathan. Antioxidant status of oxidant challenged rats treated with Bacopa monnieri leaf extract. Journal of Pharmacy Research (2011) 4(10): 3538-3539.
62 Thangarajan Sumathi, Chandrasekar Shobana, Johnson Christinal, Chandran Anusha. Protective effect of Bacopa monniera on methyl mercury-induced oxidative stress in cerebellum of rats. Cell Mol Neurobiol (2012) 32: 979-987.

---

63 Priya Verma, Poonam Singh, Behrose S Gandhi. Prophylactic efficacy of Bacopa monnieri on decabromodiphenyl ether (PBDE-209)-induced alterations in oxidative status and spatial memory in mice. Asian Journal of Pharmaceutical and Clinical Research (2013) 6(3): 242-247.

64 Chandrasekar Shobana, Thangarajan Sumathi. Studies on behavioral, biochemical, immunohistochemical and quantification of dopamine and its metabolites in the striatum of 6-hydroxy dopamine induced parkinsonism in rats – attenuation by bacoside-A, a major phytoconstituent of Bacopa monniera. International Journal of Applied Biology and Pharmaceutical Technology (2013) 4(4): 120-142.

65 G K Shinomol, R B Mythri, M M S Bharath, Muralidhara. Bacopa monnieri extract offsets rotenone-induced cytotoxicity in dopaminergic cells and oxidative impairments in mice brain. Cell Mol Neurobiol (2012) 32: 455-465.

66 George K Shinomol, Muralidhara. Bacopa monnieri modulates endogenous cytoplasmic and mitochondrial oxidative markers in prepubertal mice brain. Phytomedicine (2011) 18(4): 317-26.

67 George K Shinomol, M M Srinivas Bharath. Pretreatment with Bacopa monnieri extract offsets 3-nitropropionic acid induced mitochondrial oxidative stress and dysfunctions in the striatum of prepubertal mouse brain. Canadian Journal of Physiology and Pharmacology (2012) 90(5): 595-606.

68 Hannah P Priyanka, Preetam Bala, Sindhu Ankisettipalle, Srinivasan Thyagarajan. Bacopa monnieri and L-Deprenyl differentially enhance the activities of antioxidant enzymes and the expression of tyrosine hydroxylase and nerve growth factor via ERK 1/2 and NF-κB pathways in the spleen of female Wistar rats. Neurochemical Research (2013) 38(1): 141-152.

69 H P Priyanka, R V Singh, M Mishra, S Thyagarajan. Diverse age-related effects of Bacopa monnieri and donepezil in vitro on cytokine production, antioxidant enzyme activities, and intracellular targets in splenocytes of F344 male rats. International Immunopharmacology (2013) 15(2): 260-274.

4 – Nootropic Activity

4.1 – General

Nehlig has described cognition as follows: "The concept of cognition (from the Latin word *cognoscere* 'to know' or 'to recognize') refers to a capacity for information processing, applying knowledge and changing preferences. Cognition is a complex notion that involves at least memory, attention, executive functions, perception, language and psychomotor functions."[1] The term nootropic was coined by Giurgea[2] to refer to substances that enhance cognition. It is derived from the Greek words 'nous', meaning mind, and 'trophos', meaning to nourish[3]. Nootropics are commonly prescribed for people suffering from Alzheimer's disease, schizophrenia, stroke, attention deficit hyperactivity disorder (ADHD) and age-associated memory impairment. In addition, the use of nootropics by healthy individuals to augment normal neurocognitive functions is increasing in a number of societies[4]. Chatterjee has called the practice of intervening to improve cognition and affect in healthy individuals "cosmetic neurology"[5]. A large number of nootropics are currently available. In a recent review, Froestl and coworkers[6] classified cognitive enhancers into 19 categories based on their mechanism of action.

4.2 – Ayurveda and Cognitive Enhancers

In Ayurveda, Rasayanas are nutraceuticals that enhance vitality, rejuvenate body tissues, strengthen immunity and mitigate the ill effects associated with aging[7]. They contain essential antioxidants and modulate neuro-endocrino-immune systems[8]. Rasayanas can be organ and tissue specific. Medhya rasayanas are specific to the brain and nervous system, and have been traditionally used in Ayurveda to reduce cognitive decline as well as to preserve and enhance cognitive functions[9]. Brahmi (Bacopa monniera), Ashwagandha (Withania somnifera), Jyotishmati (Celastrus paniculatus), Shankapushpi (Clitoria ternatea), Jatamansi (Nardostachys jatamansi), Vacha (Acorus calamus) and Mandukaparni (Centella asiatica) are some of the commonly used medhya herbs.

4.3 – Animal Studies

Singh and coworkers[10] investigated the effect of an ethanol extract of Bacopa monniera (BM) on the performance of rats in various learning situations such as the shock-motivated brightness-discrimination reaction, active conditioned flight reaction and continuous avoidance response. The rats in each task group were treated with BM (40 mg/kg/day, PO) for three days before the start of testing. The rats in the active conditioned flight reaction and continuous avoidance task groups received an additional support dose every third day. The results are summarized below:

- In the shock-motivated brightness-discrimination reaction task, rats treated with BM showed better acquisition, improved retention and delayed extinction compared to the control group.
- In the active conditioned flight reaction task, rats treated with BM took less time to demonstrate a conditioned response than the control group.
- Rats treated with BM also performed better than the control group in the continuous avoidance response task. A stable baseline behavior was achieved by day 20 in the BM treated group, but not in the control group.

The authors concluded that **"our findings are in conformity with the Ayurvedic claims and indicate that Bacopa monniera can improve the performance of rats in various learning situations."**

In a subsequent investigation, Singh and coworkers[11] showed that bacosides helped mental retention capacity in rats. The shock-motivated brightness-discrimination reaction, active conditioned avoidance response and conditioned taste aversion tests were used. The results are summarized below:

- In the shock-motivated brightness-discrimination test, rats treated with bacosides (10 mg/kg, PO) 90 min before training showed a reduction in time per trial, an increase in number of positive responses and an improved learning index compared to the control group. The effect lasted for 24 hours. Relearning trials were conducted 90 min after administering a second dose of bacosides (10 mg/kg, PO), and similar learning enhancements were observed.
- For the active conditioned avoidance task, rats were treated with bacosides (10 mg/kg, PO) every other day. This group exhibited conditioned responses after 6 days, whereas the control group took more than 8 days.

- In the conditioned taste aversion response test, rats treated with bacosides showed a decrease in the intake of lithium chloride solution and an increase in sucrose solution in a dose-dependent manner compared to the control group (treated with saline). The authors concluded that "**bacosides are promising saponins having facilitatory effects on the mental retention capacity.**"

Vollala and coworkers[12] evaluated the effect of a Bacopa monniera extract on learning and memory in rats. Rats were treated with the BM extract (20, 40 or 80 mg/kg, PO) or the vehicle for 2, 4 or 6 weeks. After each treatment period, the rats were subjected to the T-maze and passive avoidance tests. The results are summarized below:

- In the T-maze test, rats treated with 20 mg/kg of BM for 2 weeks did not show an improvement in learning compared to the control group, whereas those treated with 40 or 80 mg/kg showed an improvement in their learning behavior. In the longer duration studies (4 and 6 weeks), rats treated at all BM doses showed improvement.
- In the passive avoidance test, rats treated with BM showed no significant change in behavior during exploration compared to the control group. During the retention test, rats treated with any of the administered BM doses for 4 or 6 weeks showed improvement in memory retention compared to the control group. In the 2 week study, only rats treated with 40 or 80 mg/kg of BM showed an improvement.

A similar study conducted on neonatal rat pups (10 days old) showed that treatment with a BM extract during the growth spurt period also improved learning and memory[13].

Vollala and coworkers[14] examined the effect of Bacopa monniera on the dendritic morphology of neurons in the basolateral amygdala, a region of the brain associated with a range of cognitive functions. The experimental design was similar to the one described previously[12]. Behavioral tests on rats treated with BM showed improvements in spatial learning performance and memory retention as observed previously[12]. BM treatment for 4 weeks at 40 or 80 mg/kg/day, or for 6 weeks at all administered doses resulted in an increase in dendritic length and number of branching points compared to the control group.

The authors attributed the improvement in learning and memory to the structural changes in basolateral amygdaloid neurons.

A similar study[15] was conducted using rat pups (10 days old). The results showed that treatment with BM for 4 or 6 weeks increased the dendritic length and branching of amygdaloid neurons.

Mulay and Duraiswamy[16] evaluated the nootropic effects of methanol and water extracts of Bacopa monniera (stem, leaf and whole plant). Adult albino rats (7 to 8 weeks old) were divided into a number of groups, treated with the extracts (50 or 100 mg/kg/day, PO) for 5 days, and subjected to the elevated plus maze and passive avoidance tests. Groups treated with the extracts performed better than the respective control groups in both tests. The 100 mg/kg dose was more effective than the 50 mg/kg dose. Groups treated with the methanol extracts performed better than those treated with the water extracts. The order of effectiveness of the methanol extracts was stem > leaf > whole plant. The authors concluded that **"these results clearly indicate that oral administration of BM extract improved learning and memory in rats."**

Charles and coworkers[17] investigated the effect of an ethanol extract of Bacopa monniera leaves (BMEE) on learning and memory in postnatal rats. PND-15 rats were treated with the vehicle (control) or BMEE (40 mg/kg/day, PO) from PND-15 to 29. The results are summarized below:

- The BMEE-treated group performed better in the y-maze, hole-board and passive avoidance tests during acquisition and retention trials compared to the control group, indicating learning enhancement and memory retention.
- The hindbrain homogenate of the BMEE-treated group showed increased serotonin (5-HT), tryptophan hydroxylase-2 (TPH2) mRNA, and serotonin transporter (SERT) mRNA; decreased dopamine (DA); a variation in acetylcholine (ACh); and no significant change in glutamate (Glu) compared to the control group. The level of 5-HT was higher on PND-29 and PND-37 compared to the control group, but was closer to the control group on PND-53. Similar effects were observed for TPH2 mRNA and SERT mRNA.

The authors concluded that **"BMEE treatment significantly enhances learning and retention of memory in post natal rats possibly through regulating expression of TPH 2, 5-HT metabolism and transport."**

Rajan and coworkers[18] examined the effect of a Bacopa monniera extract (BM) on hippocampus-dependent memory impairment and biochemical changes in Wistar rat pups induced by 1-(m-chlorophenyl)-biguanide (mCPBG). PND-14 pups were divided into five groups and treated as follows from PND-15 to PND-29:

Group	Treatment
1	Vehicle (i.p.) – untrained control
2	Vehicle (i.p.) – trained control
3	BM (80 mg/kg/day, PO)
4	mCPBG (10 mg/kg/day, i.p.)
5	BM (80 mg/kg/day, PO) + mCPBG (10 mg/kg/day, i.p.)

Groups 2–5 were subjected to passive avoidance tests from PND-30 to PND-32. Animals from all groups were sacrificed on PND-32, and the hippocampus was isolated for biochemical analysis. The results are summarized below:

- In the passive avoidance test, group 4 showed memory impairment compared to group 2. Groups 3 and 5 showed memory enhancement compared to groups 2 and 4, respectively.
- 5-HT_{3A} receptor expression decreased in the following order among the groups: Group 3 > Group 2 > Group 5 > Group 1 > Group 4.
- Group 3 showed increases in the levels of 5-HT, ACh, gamma aminobutyric acid (GABA) and Glu and decreases in DA compared to group 1, whereas Group 4 showed decreases in the levels of 5-HT, ACh and Glu and increases in DA as well as GABA. Group 5 showed increased levels of 5-HT, ACh and Glu and decreased DA and GABA compared to Group 4.

The authors postulated that "**the observed improvement in the hippocampal-dependent task is possibly due to combined action of serotonergic and cholinergic systems.**"

Preethi and coworkers[19] found that an extract of Bacopa monniera modulated the microRNA 124-CREB pathway and suggested a mechanism for memory enhancement. The experimental procedure was similar to the one described previously[18], with some modifications. In this investigation, the shock motivated brightness discrimination test was used for behavioral assessment. Rats were sacrificed after behavioral testing, and the hippocampus was removed for biochemical analysis. The shock motivated brightness discrimination task showed that the treatment of rat pups with BM enhanced memory, and treatment with mCPBG impaired memory. Administering BM to the mCPBG-treated rats reduced the impairment of memory. Results of the biochemical analysis are summarized below (Table 4.1):

Assay	mCPBG compared to Control	mCPBG + BME compared to mCPBG	BME compared to Control
dicer mRNA, DICER, AGO2, Pre miR-124 expression	Upregulated	Downregulated	Downregulated
Ago2 mRNA	Similar	Downregulated	Downregulated
Creb 1 mRNA, P-CREB 1, PSD-95	Similar	Upregulated	Upregulated
Total-CREB 1	Lower	Higher	Higher

Table 4.1: Effects of BME, mCPBG, mCPBG+BME on expressions of dicer, Ago2, pre-miR-124 and Creb1 mRNA; levels of DICER and AGO2; and expression patterns of P-CREB 1 and PSD-95

The authors suggested that BME might enhance synaptic plasticity via the microRNA 124-CREB pathway.

Vohora and coworkers[20] investigated the effect of an ethanol extract of Bacopa monniera on the cognitive deficit induced by Phenytoin (PHT, an anticonvulsant drug) in mice. Treatment of mice with PHT (25 mg/kg/day, PO) for 14 days provided full protection from maximal electroshock seizures (MES), but caused cognitive impairment. Treatment of mice with PHT (25 mg/kg/day, PO) for 7 days followed by treatment with PHT (25 mg/kg/day, PO) + BM (40 mg/kg/day, PO) for the next 7 days provided full protection from MES, with less cognitive impairment. The authors concluded that **"BM reduces PHT-induced cognitive deficits without affecting its anticonvulsant efficacy."**

Deval and coworkers[21] found that Bacopa monniera reduced the cognitive deficit induced by topiramate (TP) without diminishing TP's anticonvulsant efficacy in the pentylene tetrazole (PTZ) and MES models. The authors suggested that BM **"can be used as an add on therapy with other anticonvulsant drugs to reduce cognitive impairment."**

Das and coworkers[22] evaluated the antidementic and anticholinesterase activities of Bacopa monniera (BM) and Ginkgo biloba (GB) in adult male Swiss mice treated with scopolamine. Male Swiss mice were treated with the vehicle, a BM extract (30 mg/kg) or a GB extract (15-60 mg/kg) daily for 7 days. Scopolamine (3 mg/kg, i.p.) was administered to the animals on day 7. A group of animals that was not treated with the extract or scopolamine was used as a control. Animals from each group were subjected to the passive avoidance test on days 7 and 8. The scopolamine-only group showed a cognitive deficit compared to the control group in the passive avoidance task. The BM + scopolamine and GB + scopolamine groups showed less cognitive impairment compared to the scopolamine-only group, indicating the antidementic activities of the herbs.

The effect of BM and GB on AChE activity was determined in vitro. A homogenate of whole mouse brain was incubated with BM or GB (10-1000 μg/50 mL). Both herbs showed dose-dependent inhibition of AChE. Ginkgo biloba was more effective (IC_{50} = 268.33 μg) than Bacopa monniera. None of the concentrations of Bacopa monniera used were able to inhibit 50% AChE.

The authors concluded that **"the extract of G. biloba and B. monniera have potent cognitive enhancing property with different mechanisms of action."**

Kasture and coworkers[23] evaluated the nootropic activity of BacoMind in normal and amnesic rats. BacoMind is an extract of Bacopa monniera containing a number of bioactive components. Amnesia was induced by the administration of scopolamine. In the elevated plus maze, passive shock avoidance and object recognition tests, rats treated with scopolamine (0.3 mg/kg, i.p.) showed impairment of learning and memory compared to the control group. Rats treated with scopolamine (0.3 mg/kg, i.p.) followed by BacoMind (60 mg/kg/day, PO, 7 days) showed less impairment of learning and memory than the scopolamine-only group. All three tests showed nootropic activity of BacoMind in amnesic rats, whereas in normal rats, only the passive avoidance and object recognition models indicated nootropic activity.

Charles and coworkers[24] examined the effect of a Bacopa monniera extract (BME) on contextual-associative learning deficits induced by D-galactose in rats. D-galactose has been known to accelerate the aging process in rodents. Wistar rats (three months old) treated with D-galactose developed impairment of contextual associative learning and showed the following biochemical changes compared to the control group:

- Increased serum advanced glycation end product
- Decreased Nuclear transcription factor 2 (Nrf2) expression, SOD, GPx and 5-HT (hippocampus)
- Suppression of some synaptic protein expression

Rats treated with D-galactose and BME showed improved contextual associative learning and a reversal of these biochemical changes compared to the D-galactose-only group. The authors concluded that **"BME treatment attenuates D-galactose induced brain aging and regulates the level of antioxidant enzymes [and] Nrf2 expression."**

Dwivedi and coworkers[25] showed that Bacopa monniera improved memory dysfunction induced by intracerebroventricularly administered okadaic acid in rats.

Achliya and coworkers[26] evaluated the effect of an alcoholic extract of Bacopa monniera (BM) and Brahmi Ghrita (BG, a polyherbal formulation) on learning and memory in rats and mice.

In the elevated plus maze task, rats treated with BM (40 mg/kg, PO) or BG (100 mg/kg, PO) showed enhancement of learning and memory compared to the control group. In the Morris water maze test, rats treated with BG (100 mg/kg, PO) showed enhancement of spatial memory compared to the control group, whereas BM (40 mg/kg, PO) had no significant effect.

Joshi and Parle[27] evaluated the nootropic effect of Brahmi rasayana (BR) as well as its effect on whole brain AChE activity in young (8 weeks) and aged (28 weeks) mice. BR is a polyherbal formulation that contains leaves of Bacopa monniera. Piracetam (a standard nootropic agent) was used for comparison. The results are summarized below:

- The elevated plus maze test showed impairment of learning and memory in aged mice compared to young mice. Mice (young and old) treated with BR (100 or 200 mg/kg/day, PO) for 8 days showed enhancement of learning and memory compared to the corresponding control group. Treating mice with piracetam (200 mg/kg/day, i.p.) for 8 days showed similar effects to treatment with BR. Young mice injected with scopolamine (0.4 mg/kg, i.p.) showed impairment of learning and memory compared to the control group. Young mice treated with BR (100 or 200 mg/kg/day, PO) for 8 days and then injected with scopolamine (0.4 mg/kg, i.p.) showed enhancement of learning and memory compared to the scopolamine-only group.
- The passive avoidance test showed impairment of memory in aged mice compared to young mice. Mice (young and old) treated with BR (100 or 200 mg/kg/day, PO) for 8 days showed enhancement of memory compared to the corresponding control group. Young mice injected with scopolamine (0.4 mg/kg, i.p.) showed impairment of memory compared to the control group. Young mice treated with BR (200 mg/kg/day, PO) for 8 days and then

injected with scopolamine (0.4 mg/kg i.p.) showed enhancement of memory compared to the scopolamine-only group.

- Aged mice treated with BR (100 or 200 mg/kg/day, PO) and then with phenytoin (12 mg/kg, PO) showed reduced levels of AChE activity in the brain compared to the phenytoin-only group.

The authors stated that "**BR might prove to be a useful memory restorative agent in the treatment of dementia seen in elderly.**"

A number of other polyherbal formulations have also shown nootropic effects in rats/mice[28-32].

Kamkaew and coworkers[33] reported that intravenous administration of BM (20-60 mg/kg) to anesthetized rats decreased systolic and diastolic pressure without affecting heart rate.

A subsequent study[34] investigated the effect of an ethanol extract of Bacopa monniera (BM) on cerebral blood flow (CBF) in rats. Ginkgo biloba (GB) and donepezil were also examined for comparison. Wistar rats were treated with BM (40 mg/kg), GB (60 mg/kg) or donepezil (1 mg/kg) for 8 weeks. The BM and GB groups respectively showed 25% and 29% increases in CBF compared to the control group, whereas the donepezil group did not show significant change. The BM group did not show any effect on blood pressure compared to the control group. Intravenous acute infusion of BM showed a decrease in diastolic pressure (31 mm Hg) and a corresponding decrease in CBF (15%). The authors stated that "**increased CBF with B. monnieri may account for its reported procognitive effect and its further exploration as an alternative nootropic drug is worthwhile.**"

4.4 – Clinical Trials

Sharma and coworkers[35] showed that Bacopa monniera improved the mental capacities of children. In a single-blind study, 40 elementary school children (6-8 years old) were placed into a treatment (n=20) or placebo group (n=20). The children in the treatment group received one teaspoon of syrup (350 mg of Bacopa monniera) thrice a day for three months. Psychological tests to evaluate visual motor function, perceptual abilities and memory span were administered to all participants before and after treatment. Children in the treatment group showed improvement, particularly in visual motor function and memory. Children in the placebo group did not show significant improvements in any categories.

Abhang[36] evaluated the effects of a special preparation of Brahmi known as Sukshma (micro) Brahmi on various mental functions in boys (10-13 years old) of average intelligence as measured on IQ tests. Students from two classes of 7th standard were selected for the study. They were evaluated using the following tests:

- Standard Progressive Test (a general intelligence test)
- Budhimapam Kasoti (a battery of mostly verbal and a few numerical tests)
- Arithmetic test
- Memory test
- Reaction time test

One class (n=47) was given Sukshma Brahmi twice daily for 9 months, and the other class (n=53) was given a placebo. The students were retested after the treatment, using the same tests as before. After the treatment, students in the Sukshma Brahmi group performed better in the memory test, arithmetic test and four subsets of Budhimapam Kasoti, whereas those given the placebo did not show significant improvements in these tests.

Kaur and coworkers[37] evaluated an Ayurvedic formulation containing Bacopa monniera for its effect on attention, concentration and memory in school age children of normal intelligence. Fifty school children (22 boys and 28 girls) between the ages of 10 and 18 (mean age 11.85) were selected for the study. Tests were administered to evaluate attention, concentration and memory. After baseline testing, subjects were treated with the Ayurvedic formulation at 10 g/day for 6 weeks, and then retested. After a washout period of 3 months, subjects were treated with a placebo at 10 g/day for 6 weeks, and then retested. After treatment, the Ayurvedic formulation subjects showed a decrease in reaction time (auditory and visual) compared to the baseline, indicating improvement in attention. No significant changes in concentration or memory were observed. In the placebo group, no significant change in the scores of any of the three parameters was observed.

Usha and coworkers[38] conducted an open labeled clinical trial to evaluate the cognitive effect of BacoMind, an extract of Bacopa monniera, in children considered slow learners. A total of 28 healthy children (13 males and 15 females) with an IQ of 70-90 participated in the study. Each participant received a capsule of BacoMind (225 mg) daily for four months. After treatment, the participants improved in working memory, logical memory, memory related to personal life, visual memory and auditory memory.

In a placebo-controlled double-blind trial, Upadhyay and coworkers[39] evaluated the efficacy of Mentat, a polyherbal formulation containing Bacopa monniera, in children with learning disabilities. Healthy students (11-16 years old) who had poorly performed at school but had potential for better performance (IQ 90), were treated with Mentat for six months. Children who received Mentat showed improved memory, attention and concentration.

Nathan and coworkers[40] conducted a double-blind, placebo-controlled study to evaluate the effect of the acute administration of Bacopa monniera on cognitive functions in healthy normal subjects. A group of healthy volunteers consisting of 11 males (18-60 years old) and 27 females (18-53 years old) were randomly assigned to one of two groups: Bacopa or placebo. Neuropsychological tests were administered to evaluate attention, working and short-term memory, verbal learning, memory consolidation, executive processes, planning and problem solving, information processing speed, motor responsiveness and decision making. Subjects in the Bacopa group received 300 mg of an alcoholic extract of Bacopa monniera. Two hours later, the subjects were retested. Neither group showed significant changes in any of the parameters tested.

A similar study was done by Maher and coworkers[41] to evaluate the effects of a combined administration of Ginkgo biloba (GB) and Bacopa monniera (BM) on cognitive functions. Subjects were treated with a single dose of placebo or a dose of an alcoholic extract of BM (300 mg) and GB (120 mg). Cognitive testing was conducted before treatment and after 90 and 180 min of treatment. There were no significant changes in any of the parameters.

Stough and coworkers[42] examined the effect of chronic administration of Bacopa monniera on cognitive functions in healthy subjects. In a double-blind placebo-controlled trial, a group of 46 healthy volunteers (18-60 years old) consisting of 11 males and 35 females were randomly assigned to one of two groups: Bacopa (n=23) or placebo (n=23). Subjects in the Bacopa group were required to take two capsules per day for 12 weeks. Each capsule contained 150 mg of Bacopa monniera extract (KeenMind). All of the subjects were evaluated with a battery of well-validated neuropsychological tests at three time periods: prior to the commencement of the treatment; five weeks into the treatment; and at the end of the treatment. The Bacopa group showed improvements in the speed of visual information processing, verbal learning and memory consolidation as well as decreased anxiety compared to the placebo group. Considerable improvements were observed only after 12 weeks of treatment, indicating the necessity of chronic administration to elicit therapeutic effects. The investigators concluded that **"B. monniera may improve higher order cognitive processes that are critically dependent on the input of information from our environment such as learning and memory."**

Roodenrys and coworkers[43] investigated the effect of chronic administration of Bacopa monniera on memory. In a double-blind, randomized, placebo-controlled trial, 76 healthy volunteers (40-65 years old) were assigned to a Bacopa (n=37) or placebo (n=39) group. Subjects in the Bacopa group were required to take one capsule of Bacopa monniera daily (300 mg/day for persons under 90 kg; 450 mg/day for persons above 90 kg). All of the subjects were tested to assess attention, memory and psychological state prior to the commencement of the treatment, at the end of treatment and six weeks after the treatment. The Bacopa monniera group showed improvement on a task requiring retention of new information compared to the placebo group. It was suggested that this effect was probably due to less loss of information from memory rather than any difference in the rate of acquisition of information. No significant change between the groups was observed in attention, short-term memory, working memory and the retrieval of information from long-term memory. Also, there were no significant differences in subjective measures of psychological state (depression, anxiety and stress) and everyday memory functions.

Nathan and coworkers[44] evaluated the combined effect of Bacopa monniera and Ginkgo biloba on cognitive functions in healthy subjects. In a double-blind placebo-controlled trial, 85 healthy subjects (34 males and 51 females) between 19-68 years of age (mean age 41.8) were randomly placed in a placebo or Ginkgo biloba-Bacopa monniera group. Subjects in the placebo group were required to take two placebo tablets per day for 28 days, whereas those in the Ginkgo biloba–Bacopa monniera group were given two tablets of Ginkgo biloba-Bacopa monniera for 28 days. Each tablet of Ginkgo biloba-Bacopa monniera contained a Ginkgo biloba extract (equivalent to 3 g dry plant) and a Bacopa monniera extract (equivalent to 3 g dry plant). The subjects were evaluated prior to the commencement of treatment, 2 weeks into treatment and at the end of 4 weeks of treatment. The Ginkgo biloba-Bacopa monniera group showed no significant change compared to the placebo on any of the cognitive functions tested including attention, short-term and working memory, verbal learning, memory consolidation, executive processes, planning and problem solving, information processing speed, motor responsiveness and decision making.

Stough and coworkers[45] examined the nootropic effects of Bacopa monniera in healthy subjects after 90 days of treatment. In a double-blind placebo-controlled trial, 107 healthy volunteers (18-60 years old) were randomly placed in either a Bacopa or placebo group. Subjects in the Bacopa group were required to take two capsules of Bacopa monniera per day for 90 days. Each capsule contained 150 mg of a Bacopa monniera extract (KeenMind). Cognitive factors such as secondary memory, working memory, speed of memory, speed of attention, accuracy of attention and rapid visual information processing were assessed before and after treatment. 62 participants completed the trial. The Bacopa treatment improved performance on working memory, especially spatial working memory. Also, the number of false positives recorded in the rapid visual information task was reduced. The Bacopa group also showed improvement in a number of other areas, but the changes were not significant.

A comparative study of the psychomotor effects of Bacopa monniera and caffeine on healthy male subjects was conducted by Raina and coworkers[46]. Forty male medical students (25 ± 5 years) were randomly placed in either a Bacopa or caffeine group. Each subject in the Bacopa group was given 250 mg of Bacopa monniera twice a day for 16 weeks. The caffeine group received 100 mg of caffeine twice a day for the same period. The subjects were evaluated on a broad range of perceptual, motor and intellectual functions prior to the commencement of the study, and at frequent intervals afterwards. The Bacopa group did better in a number of tasks, particularly the multiple choice reaction time task, critical flicker fusion threshold task, digit cancellation task, and mental arithmetic test. The caffeine group performed better in the memory test. The authors concluded that "**Brahmi can prove to be a supplement of the utmost utility to improve cognitive functions.**"

Recently, Sathyanarayan and coworkers[47] showed that the chronic administration of Brahmi had no effect on cognitive function and anxiety in healthy subjects. In a randomized double-blind, placebo-controlled trial, 72 healthy volunteers in the age group 35-60 were randomly assigned to a placebo or Bacopa group. Each subject was instructed to consume two capsules a day (Placebo or Bacopa monniera) for 12 weeks. Each capsule of Bacopa monniera contained 225 mg of BacoMind. Tests were administered to evaluate verbal learning and memory, inspection time, attention and interference, and anxiety before and after treatment. 66 subjects (33 from each group) completed the study. No significant differences were found between the two groups on any of the cognitive and anxiety measures.

Downey and coworkers[48] conducted a double-blind, placebo-controlled trial to evaluate the acute effects of a Bacopa monniera extract on cognitive functions in healthy subjects. The study was conducted with 24 healthy volunteers (4 males and 20 females) in the age group 18-56 (mean age=25.25). Each participant was required to attend one practice session and three study sessions that were conducted a week apart. In the practice session, the participants were introduced to the test battery and procedures that would be carried out during the study visits. The cognitive demand battery (CDB) included a stress and mental fatigue visual analogue scale (VAS), two serial subtraction tasks (serial threes and serial sevens) and a rapid visual information processing task RVIP). Blood pressure was also measured. In the first study session, participants completed one cycle of CDB and their blood pressure was measured to establish baseline values. The participants were then given a placebo or KeenMind (320 or 640 mg). Randomization was performed in the distribution of capsules. Subjects received each type of treatment only once during the three study visits. After 2 hours of treatment, the subjects completed a series of six CDB cycles. An assessment of participants' ratings of stress and fatigue was done and their blood pressure was measured. The same procedure was followed during the next two study visits. No significant difference in RVIP or blood pressure was observed between the groups. The KeenMind (320 mg) group showed an improvement in performance on CDB at the first, second and fourth repetition.

Calabrese and coworkers[49] investigated the effect of Bacopa monniera on cognitive functions in elderly persons. In a double-blind placebo-controlled clinical trial, 54 healthy volunteers (over 65 years old) with a mean age of 73.5 underwent a six week placebo run-in and were then randomly placed in either a Bacopa or placebo group. Each subject in the Bacopa group received a tablet of Bacopa monniera once daily for 12 weeks. Each tablet contained 300 g of a proprietary extract. The subjects were evaluated on various cognitive functions as well as on depression, anxiety and blood pressure at the beginning of the placebo run-in, at six weeks (commencement of treatment), at 12 weeks (first follow up), and at 18 weeks (completion of treatment). The Bacopa group showed improvement in delayed recall memory and Stroop task performance (ability to ignore irrelevant information), whereas the placebo group did not show much improvement. The Bacopa group showed decreased depression, anxiety and heart rate, whereas the placebo group showed an increase in all three.

Morgan and Stevens[50] evaluated the effectiveness of Bacopa monniera at enhancing memory in healthy older persons. In a double-blind placebo-controlled trial, a group of 98 healthy volunteers (55-86 years old) were randomly assigned to a Bacopa or placebo group. Each subject in the Bacopa group was given tablets containing a special extract of Bacopa monniera with instructions to take one tablet per day for 12 weeks. Each tablet contained 300 mg of the extract. All of the subjects were evaluated on auditory verbal memory, visuospatial memory and subjective memory before commencement and after completion of the treatment. 81 participants completed the study. The Bacopa group showed improvements in memory acquisition and retention.

Peth-Nui and coworkers[51] studied the effect of Bacopa monniera on attention, cognitive processing, working memory and cholinergic and monoaminergic functions in healthy elderly persons. In a double-blind placebo-controlled trial, 60 healthy elderly volunteers (mean age=62.62) were randomly divided into three groups: placebo, Bacopa 300 and Bacopa 600. Based on their group, each participant was given a tablet of placebo or a tablet containing 300 or 600 mg of a proprietary Bacopa monniera extract once daily for 12 weeks. Attention, cognitive processing and working memory were evaluated before the commencement of treatment and at regular intervals till the 16th week (4 weeks after the end of treatment). The activities of AChE and MAO were determined from venous blood samples of subjects according to the same schedule as testing. The Bacopa groups (particularly Bacopa 300) showed improvements in the power and speed of attention, quality and speed of memory, and cognitive processing. The Bacopa groups also showed decreased AChE activity and no significant change in MAO activity.

Barbhaiya and coworkers[52] examined the effect of BacoMind on cognitive functions in elderly persons. In a randomized, double-blind, placebo-controlled trial, 65 individuals (42 males and 22 females) in the age group 50-75 (mean age=65) were randomly assigned to a placebo or BacoMind group. The subjects had memory impairment for at least one year. Each subject received a capsule of placebo or BacoMind (450 mg) once daily for 12 weeks. Pre- and post-tests confirmed that BacoMind (450 mg) treatment improved cognitive functions such as attention and verbal memory.

Hingorani and coworkers[53] examined the effect of an ethanol extract of Bacopa monniera on various cognitive functions in healthy subjects. Twenty healthy individuals in the age group 60-75 were administered a capsule of the extract (300 mg) or placebo once daily for 12 weeks. Standard cognitive tests were administered at baseline, 12 and 16 weeks. The extract treated group showed improvements in short-term memory, processing speed, attention and depression compared to the placebo group. The improvements were observed even at 16 weeks, four weeks after the completion of treatment.

Raghav and coworkers[54] studied the effect of Bacopa monniera on persons with age-associated memory impairment (AAMI). In a double-blind randomized placebo-controlled trial, 40 subjects with AAMI and without any evidence of dementia or psychiatric disorder were assigned to a placebo (n=20) or Bacopa group (n=20). Based on their group, each subject was given a placebo or 125 mg of an ethanol extract of Bacopa monniera twice daily for 12 weeks. Both groups were treated afterwards with a placebo for another 4 weeks. The subjects were evaluated for various cognitive functions before the commencement of treatment and at frequent intervals for

16 weeks. Out of the 40 participants, 18 in the Bacopa group and 17 in the placebo group completed the study. The Bacopa group showed improvements in mental control, logical memory and paired associate learning at the end of the 12th week, which was sustained in the 13th to 16th weeks.

In a systematic review of several randomized, controlled human clinical trials, Pase and coworkers[55] stated that "**Bacopa is efficacious in improving the learning and free recall of information. This suggests that Bacopa monniera could potentially be clinically prescribed as a memory enhancer**". However, they also pointed out that "**Research into cognitive-enhancing effects of Bacopa is still in its infancy, with future research required to explore the cognitive enhancing effects of Bacopa monniera at different dosage, over longer supplementation periods and in specified populations.**"

Kongkeaw and coworkers[56] conducted a meta-analysis of randomized controlled trials on the cognitive effects of Bacopa monniera extract and concluded that Bacopa monniera may be beneficial in improving cognitive function in the attention domain, especially speed of attention.

Neale and coworkers[57] compared the cognitive enhancing effect of Bacopa monniera, Panax ginseng and modafinil using published clinical studies. The highest effect sizes for cognitive outcomes were 0.77 for modafinil (visuospatial memory accuracy), 0.86 for ginseng (simple reaction time) and 0.95 for Bacopa (delayed word recall).

References

1 A Nehlig. Is caffeine a cognitive enhancer? Journal of Alzheimer's Disease (2010) 20: S85-S94.

2 C Giurgea. Pharmacology of integrative activity of the brain. Attempt at nootropic concept in psychopharmacolgy. Actual Pharmacology (Paris) (1972) 25: 115-116.

3 Arthur Saniotis. Remaking homo: ethical issues on future human enhancement. Ethics in Science and Environmental Politics (2013) 13:15-21.

4 Martha J Farah, Judy Illes, Robert Cook-Deegan, Howard Gardner, Eric Kandel, Patricia King, Eric Parens, Barbara Sahakian, Paul Root Wolpe. Neurocognitive enhancement: what can we do and what should we do? Nature Reviews, Neuroscience (2004) 5: 421-425.

5 Anjan Chatterjee. Cosmetic neurology and cosmetic surgery: parallels, predictions and challenges. Cambridge Quarterly of Healthcare Ethics (2007) 16: 129-137.

6 Wolfgang Froestl, Andreas Muhs, Andrea Pfeifer. Cognitive enhancers (nootropics) part 1: drugs interacting with receptors. Journal of Alzheimer's Disease (2012) 32: 793-887.

7 R K Sharma and Bhagwan Dash. Caraka Samhita (text with English

translation and critical exposition based on Cakrapani Datta's Ayurveda Dipika) volume 3. Chowkhamba Sanskrit Series Office, Varanasi, India, Reprint 2007

8 Manish K Pandit. Neuroprotective properties of some Indian medicinal plants. International Journal of Pharmaceutical & Biological Archives (2011) 2(5): 1374-1379.

9 Ram Harsh Singh, K Narasimhamurthy, Girish Singh. Neuronutrient impact of Ayurvedic rasayana therapy in brain aging. Biogerontology (2008) 9: 369-374.

10 H K Singh, B N Dhawan. Effect of Bacopa monniera Linn. (Brahmi) extract on avoidance responses in rat. Journal of Ethnopharmacology (1982) 5: 205-214.

11 H K Singh, R P Rastogi, R C Srimal, B N Dhawan. Effect of bacosides A and B on avoidance responses in rats. Phytotherapy Research (1988) 2(2): 70-75.

12 Venkata Ramana Vollala, Subramanya Upadhya, Satheesha Nayak. Effect of Bacopa monniera Linn. (Brahmi) extract on learning and memory in rats: a behavioral study. Journal of Veterinary Behavior (2010) 5: 69-74.

13 V R Vollala, S Upadhya, S Nayak. Learning and memory-enhancing effect of Bacopa monniera in neonatal rats. Bratisl Lek Listy (2011) 112(12): 663-669.

14 V Ramana Vollala, S Upadhya, S Nayak. Enhancement of basolateral amygdaloid neuronal dendritic arborization following Bacopa monniera extract treatment in adult rats. Clinics (Sao Paulo) (2011) 66(4): 663-671.

15 V R Vollala, S Upadhya, S Nayak. Enhanced dendritic arborization of amygdala neurons during growth spurt periods in rats orally intubated with Bacopa monniera extract. Anat Sci Int (2011) 86(4): 179-188.

16 S S Mulay, B Duraiswamy. Nootropic Studies on leaf and stem of Bacopa monnieri (Linn). Pharmacologyonline (2011) 1: 1144-1152.

17 P D Charles, G Ambigapathy, P Geraldine, M A Akbarsha, K E Rajan. Bacopa monniera leaf extract up-regulates tryptophan hydroxlase (TPH2) and serotonin transporter (SERT) expression: implications in memory formation. J Ethnopharmacology (2011) 134(1): 55-61.

18 Koilmani Emmanuvel Rajan, Hemant K Singh, Arunagiri Parkavi, Prisila Dulcy Charles. Attenuation of 1-(m-chlorophenyl)-biguanide induced hippocampus-dependent memory impairment by a standardized extract of Bacopa monniera (BESEB CDRI-08). Neurochem Res (2011) 36: 2136-2144.

19 Jayakumar Preethi, Hemant K Singh, Prisila Dulcy Charles, Koilmani Emmanuvel Rajan. Participation of microRNA 124-CREB pathway: a parallel memory enhancing mechanism of standardised extract of Bacopa monniera (BESEB CDRI-08). Neurochem Res (2012) 37(10): 2167-77.

20 Divya Vohora, S N Pal, K K Pillai. Protection from phenytoin-induced cognitive deficit by Bacopa monniera, a reputed Indian nootropic plant. Journal of Ethnopharmacology (2000) 71: 383-390.

21 K Deval, S Vaibhav, K L Krishna. Effect of Bacopa on memory deficit produced by chronic administration of topiramate in rats. Int J Pharma (2011) 1(2): 118-124.

22 Amitava Das, Girja Shankar, Chandishwar Nath, Raghawendra Pal, Satyawan

Singh, Hemant K Singh. A comparative study in rodents of standardized extracts of Bacopa monniera and Ginkgo biloba anticholinesterase and cognitive enhancing activities. Pharmacology, Biochemistry and Behavior (2002) 73: 893-900.

23 S B Kasture, V S Kasture, A J Joshua, A Damodaran, A Amit. Nootropic activity of BacoMind™, an enriched phytochemical composition from Bacopa monnieri. Journal of Natural Remedies (2007) 7(1): 166-173.

24 Prisila Dulcy Charles, Hemant K Singh, Jayakumar Preethi, Koilmani Emmanuvel Rajan. Standardized extract of Bacopa monniera (BESEB CDRI-08) attenuates contextual associative learning deficits in the aging rat's brain induced by D-galactose. Journal of Neuroscience Research (2012) 90: 2053-2064.

25 Subhash Dwivedi, Rajasekar Nagarajan, Kashif Hanif, Hefazat Hussain Siddiqui, Chandishwar Nath, Rakesh Shukla. Standardized extract of Bacopa monniera attenuates okadaic acid induced memory dysfunction in rats: effect on Nrf2 pathway. Evidence-Based Complementary and Alternative Medicine. Volume 2013, Article ID 294501, 18 pages.

26 Girish S Achliya, U Barabde, S Wadodkar, A Dorle. Effect of Brahmi Ghrita, an polyherbal formulation on learning and memory paradigms in experimental animals. Indian J Pharmacology (2004) 36(3): 159-162.

27 Hanumanthachar Joshi, Milind Parle. Brahmi rasayana improves learning and memory in mice. eCAM (2006) 3(1): 79-85.

28 S K Bhattacharya. Nootropic effect of BR-16A (Mentat), a psychotropic herbal formulation, on cognitive deficits induced by prenatal undernutrition, postnatal environmental impoverishment and hypoxia in rats. Indian J. Exp. Biol. (1994) 32(1): 31-36.

29 Chittaranjan Andrade, B V Venkataraman, Naga Rani. BR-16A enhances learning in Sprague-Dawley rats. Archives Indian Psychiat. (1995) 2(1): 42-45.

30 S S Handu, V K Bhargava. Effect of BR-16A (Mentat) on cognitive deficits in aluminum-treated and aged rats. Indian Journal of Pharmacology (1997) 29(4): 258-261.

31 Poonam Yadav, Vaibhav Uplanchiwar, Avinash Gahane, Anuj Modi, Umesh Telrandhe, Bheemachari. Nootropic activity of L-33 – a polyherbal formulation. Pharmacologyonline (2010) 2: 818-827.

32 S Uma, S Kavimani, K V Raman. Effect of saraswatarishta on learning and memory. International Journal of Phytopharmacology (2010) 1(1): 15-19.

33 N Kamkaew, C N Scholfield, K Ingkaninan, P Maneesai, H C Parkington, M Tare, K Chootip. Bacopa monnieri and its constituents is hypotensive in anaesthetized rats and vasodilator in various artery types. Journal of Ethnopharmacology (2011) 137(1): 790-795.

34 Natakorn Kamkaew, C Norman Scholfield, Kornkanok Ingkaninan, Niwat Taepavarapruk, Krongkarn Chootip. Bacopa monnieri increases cerebral blood flow in rat independent of blood pressure. Phytotherapy Research (2012) 27(1): 135-138.

35 R Sharma, C Chaturvedi, P V Tewari. Efficacy of Bacopa monniera in revitalizing intellectual functions in children. J. Res Edu Indian Med (1987) 6(1-2): 1-10.

36 Ranjana Abhang. Study to evaluate the effect of a micro (suksma) medicine derived from Brahmi (Herpestris monniera) on students of average intelligence. J.R.A.S. (1993) 14(1-2): 10-24.

37 Bindra Ramanjit Kaur, Joglekar Adhiraj, Pandit Prasad, Rane Ajita, Moghe Vijay, Desai Shanta, Dhavale Hemangeeni, Melgiri Sudha, Kamble G. Effect of an Ayurvedic formulation on attention, concentration and memory in normal school going children. Indian Drugs (1998) 35(4): 200-203.

38 P D Usha, P Wasim, J A Joshua, P Geatharini, B Murali, A S Mayachari, K Venkateshwarlu, V S Saxena, M Deepak, A Amit. BacoMind: A cognitive enhancer in children requiring individual education programme. Journal of Pharmacology and Toxicology (2008) 3(4): 302-310.

39 S K Upadhyay, Abhijeet Saha, B D Bhatia, Kala Suhas Kulkarni. Evaluation of the efficacy of Mentat in children with learning disability: a placebo-controlled double-blind clinical trial. Neurosciences Today (2002) 6(3): 184-188.

40 P J Nathan, J Clarke, J Loyd, C W Hutchison, L Downey, C Stough. The acute effects of an extract of Bacopa monniera (Brahmi) on cognitive function in healthy normal subjects. Human Psychopharmacology Clin Exp (2001) 16: 345-351.

41 Bronya F G Maher, Con Stough, Anna Shelmerdine, Keith Wesnes, Pradeep J Nathan. The acute effects of combined administration of Ginkgo biloba and Bacopa monniera on cognitive function in humans. Human Psychopharmacology Clin Exp (2002) 17: 163-164.

42 C Stough, J Loyd, J Clarke, L A Downey, C W Hutchison, T Rodgers, P J Nathan. The chronic effects of an extract of Bacopa monniera (Brahmi) on cognitive function in healthy human subjects. Psychopharmacology (2001) 156: 481-484.

43 Steven Roodenrys, Dianne Booth, Sonia Bulzomi, Andrew Phipps, Caroline Micallef, Jaclyn Smoker. Chronic effects of Brahmi (Bacopa monnieri) on human memory. Neuropsychopharmacology (2002) 27(2): 279-281.

44 Pradeep J Nathan, Sally Tanner, Jenny Lloyd, Ben Harrison, Leah Curran, Chris Oliver, Con Stough. Effect of a combined extract of Ginkgo biloba and Bacopa monniera on cognitive function in healthy humans. Human Psychopharmacology Clin Exp (2004) 19:91-96.

45 Con Stough, Luke A Downey, Jenny Lloyd, Beata Silber, Stephanie Redman, Chris Hutchison, Keith Wesnes, Pradeep J Nathan. Examining the nootropic effect of a special extract of Bacopa monniera on human cognitive functioning: 90 day double-blind placebo-controlled randomized trial. Phytotherapy Research (2008) 22: 1629-1634.

46 R S Raina, V S Chopra, R Sharma, V Khajuria, V Sawhney, V Kapoor. The psychomotor effects of Brahmi and caffeine on healthy male volunteers. Journal of Clinical and Diagnostic Research (2009) 3(6): 1827-1835.

47 Vidya Sathyanarayanan, Tinku Thomas, Suzanne J L Einother, Rajendra Dobriyal, M K Joshi, Srinivasan Krishnamachari. Brahmi for the better? New findings challenging cognition and anti-anxiety effects of Brahmi (Bacopa monniera) in healthy adults. Psychopharmacology (2013) 227(2): 299-306.

48 Luke A Downey, James Kean, Fiona Nemeh, Angela Lau, Alex Poll,

Rebecca Gregory, Margaret Murray, Johanna Rourke, Brigit Patak, Mathew P Pase, Andrea Zangara, Justin Lomas, Andrew Scholey, Con Stough. An acute, double-blind, placebo-controlled crossover study of 320 mg and 640 mg doses of a special extract of Bacopa monnieri (CDRI 08) on sustained cognitive performance. Phytotherapy Research (2013) 27(9): 1407-13.

49 Carlo Calabrese, William L Gregory, Michael Leo, Dale Kraemer, Kerry Bone, Barry Oken. Effects of a standardized Bacopa monnieri extract on cognitive performance, anxiety and depression in the elderly: a randomized double-blind, placebo-controlled trial. The Journal of Alternative and Complimentary Medicine (2008) 14(6): 707-713.

50 Annette Morgan, John Stevens. Does Bacopa monnieri improve memory performance in older persons? Results of a randomized, placebo-controlled double-blind trial. The Journal of Alternative and Complimentary Medicine (2010) 16(7): 753-759.

51 Tatimah Peth-Nui, Jintanaporn Wattanathorn, Supaporn Muchimapura, Terdthai Tong-Un, Nawanant Piyavhatkul, Poonsri Rangseekajee, Kornkanok Ingkaninan, Sakchai Vittaya-Areekul. Effects of 12-week Bacopa monnieri consumption on attention, cognitive processing, working memory, and functions of both cholinergic and monoaminergic systems in healthy elderly volunteers. Evidence-Based Complimentary and Alternative Medicine (2012). doi: 10.1155/2012/606424

52 Harshad C Barbhaiya, Rajeshwari P Desai, Vinod S Saxena, K Pravina, P Wasim, P Geetharani, J Joshua Allan, K Venkateshwarlu, A Amit. Efficacy and tolerability of BacoMind on memory improvement in elderly participants – a double blind placebo controlled study. Journal of Pharmacology and Toxicology (2008) 3(6): 425-434.

53 L Hingorani, S Patel, B Ebersole. Sustained cognitive effects and safety of HPLC-standardized Bacopa monnieri extract: a randomized, placebo controlled clinical trial. Planta Med (2012) 78: PH22.

54 Sangeeta Raghav, Harjeet Singh, P K Dalal, J S Srivastava, O P Asthana. Randomized controlled trial of standardized Bacopa monniera extract in age-associated memory impairment. Indian Journal of Psychiatry (2006) 48: 238-242.

55 Matthew P Pase, James Kean, Jerome Sarris, Chris Neale, Andrew B Scholey, Con Stough. The cognitive-enhancing effects of Bacopa monnieri: a systematic review of randomized, controlled human clinical trials. The Journal of Alternative and Complimentary Medicine (2012) 18(7): 647-652.

56 Chuenjid Kongkeaw, Piyameth Dilokthornsakul, Phurit Thanarangsarit, Nanteetip Limpeanchob, C Norman Scholfield. Meta-analysis of randomized controlled trials on cognitive effects of Bacopa monnieri extract. Journal of Ethnopharmacology (2013) 151(1): 528-535.

57 Chris Neale, David Camfield, Jonathon Reay, Con Stough, Andrew Scholey. Cognitive effects of two nutraceuticals Ginseng and Bacopa benchmarked against modafinil: a review and comparison of effect sizes. British Journal of Clinical Pharmacology (2013) 75(3): 728-737.

5 – Antiamnesic Activity

5.1 – General

Amnesia is a condition in which memory is disturbed. The loss of memory is usually temporary, but permanent loss is also possible. Causes of amnesia include damage to the brain due to infection, stroke, head injury, degenerative disorders, extensive use of drugs/alcohol, and traumatic psychological experiences. Amnesia is also a common side effect of a number of medical treatments such as electroconvulsive therapy and benzodiazepines. Amnesia is mostly of two types - anterograde and retrograde. Anterograde amnesia is characterized by the inability to form new memories, whereas retrograde amnesia refers to the inability to recall past memories. Even with mild amnesia, people may experience difficulties with daily life.

5.2 – Experimental Evidence

The antiamnesic activity of Bacopa monniera has been demonstrated by a number of investigators using animal models.

Kishore and Singh[1] examined the effect of an alcohol extract of Bacopa monniera on experimentally induced amnesia in Swiss albino mice. Scopolamine, sodium nitrite and BN52021 (a platelet activating factor receptor antagonist) were used to induce amnesia. Learning and memory were evaluated with the Morris water maze test. The results are summarized below:

- Mice treated with the extract (30 mg/kg, i.p.) 30 minutes prior to the first acquisition trials in the Morris water maze apparatus (anterograde administration) for four consecutive days showed improved acquisition compared to the control group. Administering the extract on the fifth day (prior to the first retrieval trials) did not cause a significant performance change compared to the control group. This indicated that retrograde administration of Bacopa monniera had no effect on the retrieval of old memories.
- The Morris water maze test showed that mice injected with scopolamine (3 mg/kg, i.p.) 30 minutes prior to the first acquisition trials for four consecutive days showed impairment of memory com-

pared to the control group. This indicated that scopolamine induced anterograde amnesia. Retrograde administration of scopolamine had no effect on memory. Administering the extract to scopolamine-treated mice for four consecutive days reversed the anterograde amnesia induced by scopolamine.

- Both anterograde and retrograde administration of sodium nitrite (75 mg/kg, i.p.) induced amnesia. Treatment with the extract was effective only against anterograde amnesia, and had no effect on retrograde amnesia.
- Anterograde administration of BN52021 had no effect. Retrograde administration of BN52021 (15 mg/kg, i.p.) induced amnesia, which was successfully reversed by treatment with the extract (30 mg/kg, i.p.).

The authors suggested that improvements in acetylcholine level and hypoxic condition might have enabled the reversal of anterograde amnesia induced by scopolamine and sodium nitrite, respectively. The reversal of retrograde amnesia induced by BN52021 was attributed to the enhancement of platelet activating factor synthesis by bacosides.

Prabhakar and coworkers[2] investigated the antiamnesic effect of Bacopa monniera against diazepam-induced anterograde amnesia in male Swiss albino mice. Learning and memory were evaluated with the Morris water maze test. The results are summarized below:

- Mice treated with the extract (120 mg/kg/day, PO) for six consecutive days prior to the first acquisition trials showed performance similar to the control group. Retrograde administration of the extract (120 mg/kg, PO) on the 7th day prior to the first retrieval trials showed no significant change in performance compared to the control group. These results indicated that the extract had no effect on acquisition and retrieval in normal mice.
- Mice treated with diazepam (1.75 mg/kg/day, i.p.) for six consecutive days prior to the first acquisition trials showed memory impairment compared to the control group, indicating that diazepam induced anterograde amnesia. Mice treated with diazepam prior to the first retrieval trial on day 7 performed similar to the control group, indicating that diazepam did not induce retrograde amnesia.
- Mice treated with the extract (120 mg/kg/day, PO) followed by diazepam (1.75 mg/kg/day, i.p.) for six consecutive days prior to the first acquisition trials showed enhancement of memory com-

pared to the diazepam-only group, indicating the mitigation of diazepam-induced anterograde amnesia.

The investigators suggested the involvement of the GABAergic system in mediating the antiamnesic effect.

In a subsequent investigation, Saraf and coworkers[3] reconfirmed the antiamnesic effect of Bacopa monniera against diazepam-induced amnesia, as well as examined the effect of Bacopa monniera on downstream molecules of long term potentiation (LTP) after inducing amnesia with diazepam. Diazepam-induced amnesia in mice was accompanied by downregulation and upregulation of the following:

Downregulation	• Nitrate • Nitrite • Total nitrite • Cyclic adenosine monophosphate (cAMP) • cAMP response element binding (CREB) protein expression • Phosphodiesterase (PDE)
Upregulation	• Mitogen activated protein (MAP) kinase • Phosphorylated CREB (p CREB) • Inducible nitric oxide synthase (iNOS)
No Change	• Calmodulin

Treatment with the Bacopa monniera extract reversed the amnesia, suppressed the upregulation of MAP kinase, pCREB and iNOS, and attenuated the downregulation of nitrite. It did not affect cAMP, PDE, nitrate, or total nitrite.

Saraf and coworkers[4] investigated the effect of Bacopa monniera on scopolamine-induced amnesia in mice as well as its effect on downstream molecules of LTP after scopolamine-induced amnesia. Experiments similar to those described previously[2] were conducted. Treatment of mice with scopolamine (0.1 mg/kg, i.p.) impaired acquisition in the Morris water maze test, confirming anterograde amnesia induced by scopolamine. The brain homogenate of mice treated with scopolamine showed reduced levels of protein kinase C and iNOS compared to the control group, without significantly affecting cAMP, protein kinase A, calmodulin, MAP kinase, nitrite, CREB and pCREB. Treatment of mice with the Bacopa monniera extract (120 mg/kg, PO) along with the administration of scopolamine (0.1 mg/kg, i.p.) mitigated the amnesic effect of scopolamine, as well as improved calmodulin levels. Levels of protein kinase C and pCREB were slightly improved. The authors concluded that "**Bacopa monniera induced**

suppression of scopolamine related amnesia may be mediated by PKC and CaM."

Recently, Saraf and coworkers[5] showed that scopolamine induced both anterograde and retrograde amnesia in mice, and Bacopa monniera was able to reverse both forms of amnesia.

Saraf and coworkers[6] examined the effect of Bacopa monniera on amnesia induced by N_{ω}-nitro-L-arginine (L-NNA) and MK-801. L-NNA is a nitric oxide inhibitor and MK-801 is an N-methyl-D-aspartate (NMDA) receptor antagonist.

L-NNA (30 mg/kg, i.p.) and MK-801 (0.25 mg/kg, i.p.) were found to induce both anterograde and retrograde amnesia in mice. Treatment of mice with the Bacopa monniera extract (80 mg/kg, PO) mitigated both forms of amnesia induced by L-NNA. The extract (120 mg/kg, PO) did not mitigate either form of amnesia induced by MK-801.

The authors suggested that Bacopa monniera exerts an antiamnesic effect by relieving the NOS inhibitory effect of L-NNA, but is unable to delink MK-801 from the NMDA receptor. They postulated that the **"NOS mediated pathway plays a more dominant role in Bacopa mediated reversal of amnesia."**

Joseph and coworkers[7] showed that treating rats with BR-16A (200 mg/kg/day) for 3 weeks enhanced learning as well as provided protection from anterograde amnesia induced by electroconvulsive shocks (ECS). BR-16A is a polyherbal formulation of Brahmi.

Andrade and Chandra[8] found that treating mice with a Bacopa monniera extract (500 mg/kg/day) for 15 days attenuated ECS-induced retrograde and anterograde amnesia.

Habbu and coworkers[9] evaluated the antiamnesic activity of a Bacopa-phospholipid complex (BPC) in rodents. BPC was prepared by reacting an extract of Bacopa monniera (BE) with Lα–phosphotidylcholin. Swiss albino mice (young and old) were used in the study. Antiamnesic activity was evaluated by the elevated plus maze (EPM), Morris water maze (MWM) and passive shock avoidance (PSA) tests. Aged mice showed poor retention compared to young ones in all three models (EPM, MWM and PSA). Aged mice treated with BE or BPC showed enhanced cognition and decreased brain AChE activity compared to untreated aged mice in all of the models. BPC was more effective than BE at enhancing cognition. The blood concentrations of bacopaside I and II were higher in BPC-treated rats. The authors concluded that the better anti-amnesic efficacy of BPC **"might be due to better absorption of bacopasides from the complex."**

Yadav and coworkers[10] showed the antiamnesic effect of Brahmi Ghrita (a polyherbal formulation containing Bacopa monniera) against scopolamine-induced amnesia in rats using the elevated plus maze, passive avoidance and active avoidance tests. The effect of Brahmi Ghrita was comparable to piracetam, a standard nootropic drug.

References

1 Kamal Kishore, Manjeet Singh. Effects of bacosides, alcoholic extract of Bacopa monniera linn. (Brahmi), on experimental amnesia in mice. Indian Journal of Experimental Biology (2005) 43: 640-645.
2 Sudesh Prabhakar, Manish Kumar Saraf, Promila Pandhi, Akshay Anand. Bacopa monniera exerts antiamnesic effect on diazepam-incduced anterograde amnesia in mice. Psychopharmacology (2008) 200: 27-37.
3 M K Saraf, S Prabhakar, P Pandhi, A Anand. Bacopa monniera ameliorates amnesic effects of diazepam qualifying behavior-molecular partitioning. Neuroscience (2008) 155: 476-484.
4 Manish Kumar Saraf, Akshay Anand, Sudesh Prabhakar. Scopolamine induced amnesia is reversed by Bacopa monniera through participation of kinase-CREB pathway. Neurochem Res (2010) 35(2): 279-287.
5 Manish Kumar Saraf, Sudesh Prabhakar, Krishan Lal Khanduja, Akshay Anand. Bacopa monniera attenuates scopolamine-induced impairment of spatial memory in mice. Evidenced-Based Complementary and Alternative Medicine (2011). doi: 10.1093/ecam/neq038
6 M K Saraf, S Prabhakar, A Anand. Bacopa monniera alleviates N_{ω}-nitro-L-argnine-induced but not MK-801-induced amnesia: a mouse Morris water maze study. Neuroscience (2009) 160: 149-155.
7 Jerry Joseph, B V Venkataraman, M A Naga Rani, Chittaranjan Andrade. BR-16A protects against ECS-induced anterograde amnesia. Biological Psychiatry (1994) 36: 478-481.
8 Chittaranjan Andrade, J Suresh Chandra. Anti-amnestic properties of Brahmi and mandookaparni in a rat model. Indian Journal of Psychiatry (2006) 48(4): 232-237.
9 Prasanna Habbu, Smita Madagundi, Ramesh Kulkarni, Sagar Jadav, Rashmi Vanakudri, Venkatrao Kulkarni. Preparation and evaluation of Bacopa-phospholipid complex for antiamnesic activity in rodents. Drug Invention Today (2013) 5: 13-21.
10 Kapil Deo Yadav, K R C Reddy, Vikas Kumar. Study of Brahmi ghrta and piracetam in amnesia. Ancient Science of Life (2012) 32(1): 11-16.

6 – Effect on Alzheimer's Disease (AD)

6.1 – General

Alzheimer's disease (AD) is a fatal, progressive and irreversible neurodegenerative disorder. It is the most prevalent kind of dementia among elderly people. An estimated 36 million people worldwide are suffering from dementia. It is projected that this number could jump to 66 million by 2030 and 115 million by 2050[1]. Approximately 5.4 million people in the US have AD, and it is the fifth leading cause of death among adults 65 and older[2].

Alzheimer's disease has a slow and insidious onset. It takes many years for the various behavioral deficits to manifest. It may begin as mild forgetfulness, but the memory lapses become frequent and progress to the loss of other cognitive functions. AD patients experience difficulties communicating, learning, thinking and reasoning. The problems become severe enough to have a serious impact on daily activities, family and social life.

6.2 – Causes

The cause or causes of AD are not completely known. However, a number of risk factors have been reported[3-5], which include the following:

- Advanced age

  Advanced age is the number one known risk factor. AD is generally considered a disease of old age. The risk of developing AD doubles every five years after the age of 65. Almost half the people over the age of 85 are afflicted with AD. However, AD is not an inevitable consequence of normal aging.

- Family history and genetic factors

  Individuals who have a first degree relative (parent or sibling) with AD are at an increased risk of developing AD compared to the general population. In families where AD is highly prevalent, heredity (genetics), shared environment/lifestyle, or both may play a role. A small percentage of AD cases (<1%) is known to be caused by genetic mutations. These mutations involve the gene for the amyloid precursor protein and the genes for the presenilin 1 and presenilin 2 proteins. Individuals who inherit any one of these mutations develop AD before the age of 65, and sometimes even as early as 30. This type of AD is known as "early onset" or "younger onset" AD. In the case of "late onset" AD that develops after 65 years of age, the APOE gene is the most validated genetic susceptibility factor. The APOE gene has three common alleles - e2, e3, and e4. Everyone inherits one allele from each parent. Inheriting one or two copies of APOE e4 increases the risk of developing AD. This does not mean individuals possessing one or two APOE e4 alleles will necessarily develop AD.

- Other factors

  A number of other risk factors, such as traumatic brain injury, cardiovascular disease, diabetes and mild cognitive impairment have been reported.

6.3 - Pathological Features

The brains of patients with AD show loss of synapses and neurons as well as the two hallmark lesions - extracellular senile plaques and intracellular neurofibrillary tangles (NFTs). The senile plaques contain mainly Amyloid (Aβ) peptide, which is formed by the proteolytic cleavage of the amyloid precursor protein (APP). Soluble monomers of Aβ aggregate into oligomers, proto-fibrils and eventually amyloid fibrils. Neurofibrillary tangles are composed of abnormally hyperphosphorylated tau protein. Tau is an axonal protein that binds to microtubules and provides stability. During the course of AD, tau becomes abnormally phosphorylated, dissociates from microtubules and aggregates into paired helical filaments[6,7].

6.4 - Diagnosis

At the present time, there is no accurate and reliable laboratory test for AD. However, well established criteria are available to guide in the diagnosis, which is based on physical, psychological and neurological evaluation as well as some laboratory tests of patients suffering from dementia[8,9]. The approach is essentially a process of elimination. Doctors evaluate other causes for dementia and confirm AD by eliminating them. Intense research is going on to discover a reliable test for the early diagnosis of AD. These include biochemical markers in tissues and body fluids as well as measurements of brain volume and activity based on neuroimaging modalities[10-13]. Recently, the National Institute on Aging and the Alzheimer's Association have recommended new diagnostic criteria and guidelines for AD. The recommendations include the identification of three stages of AD and the incorporation of biomarkers[2].

6.5 – Treatment

AD is currently an incurable disease. Existing drugs are symptomatic only and have modest efficacy. FDA approved drugs for managing AD include cholinesterase inhibitors (donepezil, rivastigmine, galantamine) and an NMDA receptor antagonist (memantine). Relentless research is under way to develop disease-modifying drugs for AD. In 2011, over 80 compounds with AD-modifying properties were reported to be in clinical trials[12].

6.6 – Ayurveda and Alzheimer's disease

Alzheimer's disease is not specifically mentioned in classical Ayurvedic texts. Modern Ayurveda considers AD to be an age related disorder with vata[14]. Ayurvedic treatment of AD includes rasayana therapy with special herbal formulations. Recently, herbal remedies for AD have received a lot of attention and a number of papers have been published[14-19].

6.7 – Experimental Evidence

Bhattacharya and coworkers[20] investigated the effect a Bacopa monniera extract (BM) on the cognitive deficit and perturbation of cholinergic functions induced by colchicine and ibotenic acid in mice (animal models of AD). Colchicine was administered intracerebroventricularly (icv). Ibotenic acid was injected into the right side of the nucleus basalis magnocellularis (nbm). Adult male Wistar rats treated with colchicine (15 μg) or ibotenic acid (10 μg) showed a retention deficit compared to the control group. Also, colchicine-treated rats showed decreased ACh, activity of ChAT, and MCR binding in the frontal cortex and hippocampus compared to the control group. Rats treated with colchicine or ibotenic acid followed by BM (10 mg/kg/day, PO) for 7 or 14 days showed a reversal of these changes. The authors observed that **"the nootropic effect of BM may be, at least in part, due to reversal of perturbed cholinergic function responsible for memory deficits."**

Holcomb and coworkers[21] examined the effect of an alcoholic extract of Bacopa monniera leaves (BME) on the performance of transgenic mice in the y-maze and open field location tasks, as well as on the levels of $A\beta_{1-40}$ and $A\beta_{1-42}$ in the cortex. Transgenic PSAPP mice (PND-60) were treated with regular powdered rodent chow (transgenic control) or powdered rodent chow containing BME (40 or 160 mg/kg/day) for 2 months (short term) or 8 months (long term). The short term period corresponds to the early phase of amyloid deposition, and the long term period corresponds to the rapid increase of plaque. Non-transgenic mice were also treated in a similar manner (non-transgenic control). All of the animals were subjected to the y-maze and open field tasks during the last four days of treatment. They were then sacrificed and brain samples were removed for analysis. The results are summarized below:

- In the short-term experiment, both the transgenic and non-transgenic control groups showed a similar performance in the y-maze task. BME treatment showed no significant effect on performance. In the long-term experiment, the transgenic control group showed impairment of spatial working memory compared to the non-transgenic control group. Transgenic mice treated with BME (40 mg/kg) showed improved spatial working memory compared to the transgenic control group. In the open field locomotion test (short and long), the transgenic control group showed excess locomotion and loss of aversion to explore an exposed area compared to the non-transgenic control group. BME-treated transgenic mice showed a reversal of these changes, with the lower dose being more effective.
- In the short-term experiment, BME-treated (40 or 160 mg/kg) transgenic mice showed decreased $A\beta_{1-40}$ and $A\beta_{1-42}$ in the cortex but not in the hippocampus compared to the transgenic control group. In the long-term experiment, transgenic mice treated with BME (40 or 160 mg/kg) showed decreased $A\beta_{1-40}$ and $A\beta_{1-42}$ in the cortex compared to the transgenic control group. BME treatment at 160 mg/kg also reduced $A\beta_{1-40}$ and $A\beta_{1-42}$ in the hippocampus. In the long-term treatment, transgenic mice treated with BME (40 or 160 mg/kg) did not show significant changes in fibrillar amyloid load or plaque size compared to the transgenic control group.

The authors concluded that **"its effects to reduce amyloid levels and reverse behavior deficits in the PSAPP transgenic Alzheimer's model indicate that BME has considerable potential as a therapeutic intervention in Alzheimer's disease."**

Limpeanchob and coworkers[22] examined the effect of an alcoholic extract of Bacopa monniera (BME) on beta-amyloid- and glutamate-induced toxicity. Primary cortical cells prepared from 18 day old Sprague Dawley rat fetuses were used. The cells were incubated with 50 μM aggregated $A\beta_{25-35}$ or 4 mM glutamate with or without BME (100 μg/mL) for 48 hours. In the absence of BME, $A\beta_{25-35}$ and glutamate caused 21% and 30% cell death, respectively. In the presence of BME, only cell death induced by $A\beta_{25-35}$ was reduced. Incubation of cortical cells with $A\beta_{25-35}$ increased intracellular AChE activity. Incubation of cells with $A\beta_{25-35}$ and BME lowered AChE activity. Also, BME-treated cortical cells showed lower levels of ROS compared to untreated cells. This study additionally demonstrated the antioxidant and anti-LPO effect of BME. The authors concluded that **"overall results from the present study support the potential of Brahmi extract as a remedy to prevent memory loss in natural aging as well as an alternative remedy for neurodegenerative disorders associated with oxidative stress and amyloid-induced memory loss."**

Uabundit and coworkers[23] studied the effect of an alcoholic extract of Bacopa monniera (BME) on memory impairment and neurodegeneration in an animal model of AD. Ethylcholine aziridinium ion (AF64A), a cholinotoxin, was used to induce AD. Adult male Wistar rats were divided into four main groups and treated for 3 weeks as follows:

Group	Daily Dose (3 weeks)	Single Dose (end of week 2)
1	Vehicle (PO)	ACSF
2	Vehicle (PO)	AF64A
3	Aricept (PO)	AF64A
4	BME (20, 40 or 80 mg/kg/day, PO)	AF64A
AF64A (2 nmol/2 μL) was infused bilaterally via icv. Aricept (donepezil), an AChE inhibitor, is a standard drug for dementia.		

The animals were subjected to the Morris water maze test and then sacrificed to determine the density of surviving neurons in various subregions of the hippocampus. The results are summarized below:

- Group 2 showed a cognitive deficit compared to the control group. Groups 3 and 4 showed attenuation of the cognitive deficit induced by AF64A.
- Group 2 showed decreased neuron density in all four subregions of the hippocampus studied (CA1, CA2, CA3 and dentate gyrus) compared to group 1. Group 3 reduced the effect of AF64A in CA3 only. Group 4 at 20 mg reduced the effect in all four subregions; at 40 mg in CA1, CA2 and CA3; and at 80 mg in CA1 only.

- Group 2 showed decreased cholinergic neuron density in all four subregions. Group 3 reduced the effect of AF64A in all four subregions. Group 4 (40 mg) reduced the effect of AF64A in CA1 and CA2.

The authors concluded that "**Bacopa monniera is a valuable candidate for cognitive enhancement and neuroprotection in Alzheimer's disease.**"

Singh and coworkers[24] studied the effect of a Bacopa monniera extract on H_2O_2 and acrolein induced toxicity in the human neuroblastoma cell line SK-N-SH. SK-N-SH cells were treated with the extract (0–100 µg/mL) and after 3 h, acrolein (15 µM) or H_2O_2 (200 µM) was added. In the absence of the extract, acrolein induced 50% cell death after 24 h, whereas pretreatment with the extract (40–100 µg/mL) reduced cell death. Lactate dehydrogenase (LDH) release induced by acrolein was also reduced by pretreatment with the extract. Adding H_2O_2 to cells caused considerable cell death in the absence of the extract, whereas pretreatment with the extract (50–100 µg/mL) reduced cell death as well as LDH release.

A number of other experiments were conducted in this study to understand the mechanism of neuroprotection provided by Bacopa monniera. The authors suggested that "**in the long term, BM may be of therapeutic use in the prevention of AD as well as other age-related neurodegenerative disorders in which oxidative stress and mitochondrial dysfunctions are involved.**"

Ahirwar and coworkers[25] examined the effect of an ethanol extract of Bacopa monniera on anticholinesterase activity in various regions of the rat brain. Adult male rats were given double distilled water (control) or a BM extract (100 mg/kg/day, PO) for 15 days. BM-treated rats showed inhibition of AChE in all regions of the brain studied compared to the control group: cerebral cortex (51.6%), cerebellum (51%), pons (44.8%), thalamus (41.6%), hippocampus (38.1%), brain stem (34.3%) and striatum (24.9%). The authors suggested that "**Bacopa monniera may be a new potential resource of natural anticholinesterase compounds as a herbal alternative for AD treatment.**"

Saini and coworkers[26] investigated the effect of Bacopa monniera on colchicine-induced cognitive impairment, oxidative stress and other biochemical changes in rats. Male Wistar rats treated with colchicine (15 µg) showed the following changes compared to the control group:

- Memory impairment (elevated plus maze test)
- Increased LPO and PC (cortex and hippocampus)

- Decreased SOD, CAT, GR, GST and GSH (cortex and hippocampus)
- Decreased Na^+/K^+-ATPase (cortex and hippocampus)
- Increased AChE (cortex and hippocampus)

Rats treated with colchicine followed by BM (50 mg/kg/day, PO) for 15 days showed a reversal of these changes. The authors concluded that **"Bacopa monniera may prevent cognitive decline in AD through free radical scavenging activity, maintenance of thiol status and upregulation of antioxidant enzymes."**

Kunte and Kuna[27] studied the effect of a methanol extract of Bacopa monniera on the cognitive deficit and loss of ATPase activity (in different brain regions) induced by D-galactose and sodium nitrite in mice. Loss of ATPase activity is known to be involved in the development of neurological disorders. Male albino mice (one month old) treated with D-galactose (120 mg/kg) and sodium nitrite (90 mg/kg) for 60 days showed the following changes compared to the control group:

- Less weight gain
- Impairment of learning and memory
- Decreased levels of ATPases (Na^+/K^+, Mg^{2+} and Ca^{2+}) in the cerebral cortex, hippocampus, cerebellum, pons, medulla and spinal cord

Mice treated with D-galactose, sodium nitrite and BME (100 mg/kg) showed a reversal of these changes. Treatment with BME was started 10 days after the administration of D-galactose and sodium nitrite, and was continued for up to 180 days.

Vattananupon and coworkers[28] investigated the effect of an ethanol extract of Bacopa monniera (BM) on impairments in spatial learning and memory, as well as on the death of hippocampal CA1 neurons induced by chronic cerebral hypoperfusion in rats. Adult male Wistar rats (4 weeks old) were divided into five groups. Chronic hypoperfusion was induced in groups 2-5 using permanent bilateral common carotid artery occlusion or a modified 2-VO model. Group 1 (non-ischemic control) received the same surgical operation without the carotid artery ligation. Groups 1 and 2 (negative control) were given 1 mL of 0.9% saline for 8 weeks. Groups 3, 4 and 5 were treated with 120, 160 and 240 mg/kg of BM extract, respectively, for 8 weeks. Group 2 showed impairment of spatial learning and memory compared to group 1. The BM treated groups (3-5) showed less impairment in spatial learning and memory compared to group 2. Group 2 showed a reduction of hippocampal CA1 neurons compared to group 1.

The BM treated groups showed larger numbers of hippocampal CA1 neurons compared to groups 1 and 2.

Rastogi and coworkers[29] evaluated the potential of bacosides in delaying the harmful effects of aging and preventing age-associated pathologies like senile dementia of the Alzheimer's type (SDAT). Aged female Wistar rats (>24 months old) were treated with bacosides (200 mg/kg/day, PO) for 3 months. Untreated young rats (2-3 months old) were examined for comparison. The results are summarized below (Table 6.1):

Test/Assay	Aged rats compared to Young rats	Aged rats + BM compared to Aged rats
Passive avoidance	Memory impaired	Memory improved
Tail suspension	Depressive behavior	Less depressive behavior
Closed field	Deficit in gross behavioral activity	Improved gross behavioral activity
Lipofuscin (cortex)	Increased	Decreased
ACh, AChE, 5-HT, DA (cortex)	Decreased	Increased
LPO, LHP, PC (cortex)	Increased	Decreased
GSH, GR, SOD, CAT, GPx (cortex)	Decreased	Increased

Table 6.1: Effects of BM on age-associated pathologies

The authors concluded that "**the results of the present study suggest that bacosides may act as a potential therapeutic intervention in forestalling the deleterious effect of aging and preventing the age associated pathologies like SDAT.**"

In a subsequent investigation, Rastogi and coworkers[30] demonstrated that administering bacosides (200 mg/kg, PO) to middle-aged (17-18 months old) and aged (>24 months old) rats for 3 months inhibited the age-dependent increase of proinflammatory cytokines (IL-1β and TNF-α), iNOS protein expression, total nitrite and lipofuscin content in the cortex.

Mathew and Subramanian[31] showed in vitro that a methanol extract of Bacopa monniera prevented the aggregation of Aβ and facilitated dissociation of preformed Aβ aggregates.

In an open label, prospective, uncontrolled, non-randomized trial, Goswami and coworkers[32] showed that the Bacopa monniera treatment of geriatric patients suffering from AD improved some aspects of cognition. Fifty patients newly diagnosed with AD participated in the trial. The patients were administered the Mini Mental Stat Examination (MMSE), a widely used test of cognitive functions among the elderly. Patients were treated with 300 mg of Bacopa monniera extract twice daily for 180 days. Patients were interviewed once every 20 days. MMSE was again administered after the completion of the treatment. Participants showed improvement in the following tasks: orientation of time, place and person; attention; reading; writing; comprehension. Components such as registration, recall and design did not significantly change. Women showed more improvement in orientation, attention and language components than men did. Participants and their caregivers reported improvements in quality of life, memory power and sleep, along with less irritability and more positive behavior towards family.

References

1 Martin Prince, Renata Bryce, Cleusa Ferri. World Alzheimer Report 2011: The Benefits of Early Diagnosis and Intervention. Alzheimer's Disease International, 2011.

2 Alzheimer's Association. 2012 Alzheimer's disease facts and figures. Alzheimer's & Dementia (2012) 8(2): 131-168.

3 Nazem Bassil, George T Grossberg. Evidence-based approaches to preventing Alzheimer's disease, part 1. Primary Psychiatry (2009) 16(6): 29-37.

4 William Thies, Laura Bleiler. 2012 Alzheimer's disease facts and figures. Alzheimer's & Dementia (2012) 8: 131-168.

5 John W Williams, Brenda L Plassman, James Burke, Tracey Holsinger, Sophiya Benjamin. Preventing Alzheimer's disease and cognitive decline. Evidence Report/Technology Assessment No. 193 (2010). AHRQ Publication No 10-E005. US Department of Health and Human Services, Rockville, MD.

6 Karen Duff, Faraha Suleman. Transgenic mouse models of Alzheimer's disease: how useful have they been for therapeutic development? Briefings in Functional Genomics and Proteomics (2004) 3(1): 47-59.

7 Sethu Sankaranarayanan. Genetically modified mice models for Alzheimer's disease. Current Topics in Medicinal Chemistry (2006) 6: 609-627.

8 DSM-IV-TR: Diagnostic and statistical manual of mental disorders, fourth edition, text revision. American Psychiatric Association, Arlington, VA, 2000.

9 G McKhann, D Drachman, M Folstein, R Katzman, D Price, E M Stadlan. Clinical diagnosis of Alzheimer's disease: report of the NINCDS-ADRDA work group under the auspices of department of health and human services task force on Alzheimer's disease. Neurology (1984) 34(7): 939-44.

10 L Urbanelli, A Magini, V Ciccarone, F Trivelli, M Polidoro, B Tancini, C Emiliani. New perspectives for the diagnosis of Alzheimer's disease. Recent Patents on CNS Drug Discovery (2009) 4: 160-181.

11 Fatai K Salawu, Joel T Umar, Abdulfatai B Olokoba. Alzheimer's disease: A review of recent developments. Ann. Afr. Med. (2011) 10(2): 173-179.

12 Jeffrey L Cummings. Biomarkers in Alzheimer's disease drug development. Alzheimer's & Dementia (2011) 7: e13-e44.

13 Harald Hampel, David Prvulovic, Stefan Teipel, Frank Jessen, Christian Luckhaus, Lutz Frolich, Mathias W Riepe, Richard Dodel, Thomas Leyhe, Lars Bertram, Wolfgang Hoffmann, Frank Faltraco. The future of Alzheimer's disease: the next 10 years. Progress in Neurobiology (2011) 95: 718-728.

14 Divya Shangari Vohora, Lakshmi Chandra Mishra. "Alzheimer's disease" in Scientific Basis of Ayurvedic Therapies. Edited by Lakshmi Chandra Mishra. CRC Press, Boca Raton FL, 2004.

15 Thimmappa S Anekonda, P Hemachandra Reddy. Can herbs provide a new generation of drugs for treating Alzheimer's disease? Brain Research Reviews (2005) 50: 361-376.

16 Keyvan Dastmalchi, H J Damien Dorman, Heikki Vuorela, Raimo Hiltunen. Plants as potential sources for drug development against Alzheimer's disease. Int J Biomed Pharm Sci (2007) 1(2): 83-104.

17 Mohini Gore, Preenon Bagchi, N S Desai, Ajit Kar. Ayur-informatics: establishing an in-silico-ayurvedic medication for Alzheimer's disease. International Journal of Bioinformatics Research (2010) 2(1): 33-37.

18 Narendra Singh, B R Pandey, Pankaj Verma. An overview of phytotherapeutic approach in prevention and treatment of Alzheimer's syndrome & dementia. Int J Pharm Sci Drug Res (2011) 3(3): 162-172.

19 Rammohan V Rao, Oliver Descamps, Varghese John, Dale E Bredesen. Ayurvedic medicinal plants for Alzheimer's disease: a review. Alzheimer Research & Therapy (2012) 4: 22.

20 Salil K Bhattacharya, Ashok Kumar, Shibnath Ghosal. Effect of Bacopa monniera on animal models of Alzheimer's disease and perturbed cholinergic markers of cognition in rats. Research Communications in Pharmacology and Toxicology (1999) 4 (3 & 4): II-1 – II-22.

21 Leigh A Holcomb, Murali Krishnan Dhanasekaran, Angie R Hitt, Keith A Young, Mark Riggs, Bala V Manyam. Bacopa monniera extract reduces amyloid levels in PSAPP mice. Journal of Alzheimer's Disease (2006) 9: 243-251.

22 Nanteetip Limpeanchob, Somkiet Jaipan, Saisunee Rattanakaruna, Watoo Phrompittayarat, Kornkanok Ingkaninan. Neuroprotective effect of Bacopa monnieri on beta-amyloid-induced cell death in primary cortical culture. Journal of Ethnopharmacology (2008) 120: 112-117.

23 N Uabundit, J Wattanathorn, S Mucimapura, K Ingkaninan. Cognitive enhancement and neuroprotective effects of Bacopa monnieri in Alzheimer's disease model. Journal of Ethnopharmacology (2010) 127: 26-31.

24 Manjeet Singh, Ven Murthy, Charles Ramassamy. Modulation of hydrogen peroxide and acrolein-induced oxidative stress, mitochondrial dysfunctions

and redox regulated pathways by the Bacopa monniera extract: potential implication in Alzheimer's disease. Journal of Alzheimer's Disease (2010) 21: 229-247.

25 S Ahirwar, M Tembhre, S Gour, A Namdeo. Anticholinesterase efficacy of Bacopa monnieri against the brain regions of rat – a novel approach to therapy for Alzheimer's disease. Asian J. Exp. Sci. (2012) 26(1): 65-70.

26 N Saini, D Singh, R Sandhir. Neuroprotective effects of Bacopa monnieri in experimental model of dementia. Neurochem Res (2012) 37: 1928-1937.

27 Kalyani Bai Kunte, Yellamma Kuna. Neuroprotective effect of Bacopa monniera on memory deficits and ATPase system in Alzheimer's disease (AD) induced mice. Journal of Scientific and Innovative Research (2013) 2(4): 719-735.

28 S Vattananupon, P Chadvongvan, P Akarasereenont, S Tapechum, K Tilokskulchai, N Pakaprot. Brahmi extract attenuated spatial learning and memory impairment and cell death of rat hippocampal CA1 neurons after the 2-VO induced chronic cerebral hypoperfusion. Siriraj Med J (2013) 65: 105-111.

29 Manisha Rastogi, Rudra P Ojha, P C Prabu, B Parimala Devi, Aruna Agrawal, G P Dubey. Prevention of age-associated neurodegeneration and promotion of healthy brain ageing in female Wistar rats by long term use of bacosides. Biogerontology (2012) 13: 183-195.

30 Manisha Rastogi, Rudra P Ojha, B Parimala Devi, Aabha Aggarwal, Aruna Agrawal, G P Dubey. Amelioration of age associated neuroinflammation on long term bacosides treatment. Neurochem Res (2012) 37: 869-874.

31 Maya Mathew and Sarada Subramanian. Evaluation of the anti-amyloidogenic potential of nootropic herbal extracts in vitro. Int J Pharm Sci Res (2012) 3(11): 4276-4280.

32 Shishir Goswami, Anand Saoji, Navneet Kumar, Vijay Thawani, Meenal Tiwari, Manasi Thawani. Effect of Bacopa monnieri on cognitive functions in Alzheimer's disease patients. International Journal of Collaborative Research on Internal Medicine & Public Health (2011) 3(4): 285-293.

7 – Effect on Parkinson's Disease (PD)

7.1 – General

Parkinson's disease (PD) is a chronic, progressive neurological disorder. It is the second most prevalent neurodegenerative disorder after AD. An estimated 7-10 million people worldwide have PD and about a million of those cases are in the US[1]. Four conspicuous symptoms of PD are tremors, rigidity, bradykinesia (slowed motion) and postural instability[2]. The onset of PD is very subtle and the symptoms are not noticeable for a long period of time. As the disease progresses, individuals may experience difficulty in walking, talking and completing simple tasks. The rate of progression varies from individual to individual.

7.2 – Risk factors

Although the cause of PD is not fully understood, it is likely to involve both genetic and environmental risk factors. A number of risk factors have been identified, including the following:

- Advanced age[3,4]

  Advanced age is the strongest known risk factor of PD. It affects more than 1% of the population over the age of 60.

- Gender[1,5]

  PD is more common in men than women. Men are at higher risk (1.5x) of developing PD than women.

- Genetics[2,6-10]

  During the past two decades, significant progress has been made in the identification of distinct genetic loci responsible for inherited forms of PD. Genetic influences are significant in early-onset PD, and recent investigations have identified a number of susceptibility genes that play a role in late-onset PD.

- Environment[9-12]

Studies have shown that exposure to pesticides may increase the risk of developing PD.

7.3 – Pathological features[13-17]

Parkinson's disease develops with the progressive loss of dopamine-producing neurons in the substantia nigra area of the brain, which results in a dopamine deficiency. Dopamine plays an important role in many brain processes including voluntary movement, behavior, cognition, mood and reward. When dopaminergic neurons in the striatum are reduced below a minimum threshold, PD motor symptoms begin to appear. The presence of cytoplasmic inclusions in the surviving dopaminergic neurons called Lewy bodies, which are mainly composed of alpha-synuclein and other proteins, is also observed. The mechanism(s) of dopaminergic neuron loss is not well understood. A number of factors such as mitochondrial dysfunction, oxidative stress, altered protein handling and inflammatory change are considered to be involved.

7.4 – Diagnosis and Treatment[18-21]

At present, there are no laboratory tests for PD. Diagnosis is based on medical history, review of symptoms and neurological and physical examination. Sometimes, laboratory tests may be necessary to rule out other conditions that mimic PD. In addition, effective PD drugs may be administered and significant improvement may be used to confirm the diagnosis.

Currently, there is no cure for PD. However, symptoms can be controlled for years with medication. Drugs available for symptomatic treatment include levodopa (L-Dopa), dopamine agonists, inhibitors of enzymes that inactivate dopamine (e.g. monoamine oxidase-B and catechol-O-methyl transferase), anti-cholinergics and antiviral drugs (e.g. amantadine). Surgical procedures are available for advanced patients of PD who no longer respond to drugs.

7.5 – Ayurveda and Parkinson's disease[22-24]

In Ayurveda, neurodegenerative disorders are considered to result from vata imbalance. Among the various vata disorders, clinical features of Kampavata resemble those of PD. In Sanskrit, kampa means tremors and kampavata can be translated as "tremors due to vata imbalance". Treatment of kampavata is mainly directed at reversing the vata imbalance. The treatment includes panchakarma, physiotherapy and medicinal treatment using a wide range of drugs. Medhya rasayana herbs are commonly used.

7.6 – Experimental Evidence

Andrade and coworkers[25] found that BR-16A, a polyherbal formulation containing Brahmi and a number of other herbs, enhanced the activity of postsynaptic dopamine receptors in laboratory rats, indicating the potential of BR-16A in PD therapy. BR-16A was also tested on a 67-year-old patient suffering from PD[26]. The patient had previously received anticholinergic medication, but the treatment was discontinued due to side effects. A significant improvement in tremors was observed after one month of treatment with BR-16A, which was sustained even after six months. The patient was able to write and sign his name, drink coffee without spilling, and button his own clothing, which he could not do before treatment. However, there was no improvement in gait posture or bradykinesia. There was little difference in depression, motor dexterity and memory between pre- and post-treatment.

Hosamani and Muralidhara[27] investigated the effect of a Bacopa monniera extract on rotenone-induced oxidative stress and toxicity in Drosophila melanogaster. Rotenone is a natural pesticide and chronic exposure of some animals to rotenone has been reported to induce many key features of PD. Drosophila melanogaster (wild, Oregon K) adult male flies (8-10 days old) were used. Flies were treated with rotenone (500 μM) or rotenone+BM (0.1%) for 7 days. Major findings from this investigation are summarized below (Table 7.1):

Test/Assay	Rotenone compared to Control	Rotenone + BME compared to Rotenone
Mortality	48%	< 48%
Locomotor activity	Showed impairment	Showed less impairment
MDA, HP, PC (whole body homogenate)	Increased	Decreased
GSH (whole body homogenate)	Decreased	Increased
CAT, SOD, GST, DA (head and rest of body)	Decreased	Increased

Table 7.1: Effects of BME on rotenone-induced toxicity and oxidative stress

The authors concluded that "**dietary feeding of BM powder to Drosophila for a short duration has the propensity to attenuate rotenone induced oxidative stress owing to its antioxidative nature and its ability to modulate the activities of antioxidant defenses such as reduced GSH...**"

Shinomol and coworkers[28] investigated the effect of an ethanol extract of Bacopa monniera on rotenone-induced cytotoxicity in dopaminergic cells (in vitro) and oxidative impairment in the mouse brain (in vivo).

In vitro incubation of dopaminergic neuronal cells (N27) with rotenone (ROT) resulted in considerable cell death within 48 h, with LC_{50} and LC_{75} values of 8 and 16 μM, respectively. Pretreatment of N27 cells with BME (2-6 μg) for 24 h followed by exposure to ROT (8 or 16 μM) reduced cell death induced by ROT. N27 cells incubated with ROT showed increased ROS and HP, and decreased GSH compared to the control group. Pretreatment with BME reversed the rotenone-induced changes.

The antioxidant activity of BME was examined in vivo. Prepubertal male mice (4 weeks old) treated with ROT (1.0 mg/kg/day, i.p.) for 7 days showed the following changes in the cortex, cerebellum, hippocampus and striatum compared to the control group:

- Increased LPO, ROS, HP, PC, SOD
- Decreased GSH, CAT, GPx, GR
- Decreased AChE in the striatum; increased AChE in other areas
- Decreased BChE

Mice treated with BME (5 mg/kg/day, i.p.) and ROT for 7 days showed a reversal of these changes. The authors suggested that "**BM may be effectively exploited as a prophylactic/therapeutic adjuvant for neurodegenerative disorders involving oxidative stress.**"

Swathi and co-workers[29] investigated the effect of an alcohol extract of Bacopa monniera on glutamine (Gln) content and the activities of glutamate dehydrogenase (GDH), glutamine synthetase (GS) and glutaminase in various brain regions of rats treated with rotenone. The results are summarized below:

- Male Wistar rats treated with rotenone (2.5 mg/kg/day, i.p.), once daily for 60 days showed increases in glutaminase activity and decreases in the activities of GS and GDH as well as Gln content in various brain regions (cerebral cortex, cerebellum, midbrain and pons-medulla) compared to the control group, indicating the formation of glutamate and progression of PD.

- Rats treated with BM (180 mg/kg/day, PO) for 20 days and then with both BM and rotenone (2.5 mg/kg/day, i.p) for an additional 60 days showed decreases in glutaminase activity and increases in the activities of GS and GDH as well as Gln content in various regions of the brain compared to the rotenone-only treated group, indicating modulation of glutamate metabolism by BM.
- Treating rats with levodopa (10 mg/kg/day, PO) along with rotenone yielded results similar to BM.

The authors concluded that **"the Bacopa monneri extract effectively regulates glutamatergic hyperexcitation and can be used as an antiparkinsonian agent."**

Swathi and co-workers[30] also studied the effect of an alcohol extract of Bacopa monniera on the activities of Na^+/K^+-ATPase, Mg^{2+}-ATPase and Ca^{2+}-ATPase in various brain regions of rats treated with rotenone. The results are summarized below:

- Rats treated with rotenone (2.5 mg/kg/day, i.p), once daily for 60 days showed decreased Na^+/K^+-ATPase, Mg^{2+}-ATPase and Ca^{2+}-ATPase in the cerebral cortex, cerebellum, midbrain and pons-medulla compared to the control group, indicating impairment of energy metabolism induced by rotenone. Rats treated with BM (180 mg/kg/day, PO) for 20 days and then with both BM and rotenone (2.5 mg/kg/day, i.p) for 60 days showed increased Na^+/K^+-ATPase, Mg^{2+}-ATPase and Ca^{2+}-ATPase in these brain regions compared to the rotenone-only group.
- Treatment of rats with levodopa (10 mg/kg/day, PO) along with rotenone yielded results similar to BM.

The authors concluded that the **"ethanolic extract effectively regulated ATPase activity by decreasing oxidative stress/recovering the energy loss that has occurred due to PD and thus can be used as an antiparkinsonian agent."**

Hosamani and Muralidhara[31] examined the prophylactic treatment of adult Drosophila melanogaster with Bacopa monniera leaf powder on paraquat (PQ, a widely used herbicide) induced lethality, oxidative stress and mitochondrial dysfunction. Drosophila melanogaster (wild, Oregon K) adult male flies (8-10 days old) were used in this study. The results are summarized below:

- Flies exposed to PQ (40 mM in 5% sucrose solution) for 48 hours suffered 50% mortality, whereas those fed with a BM (0.1%) supplemented diet for 7 days and then exposed to PQ (40 mM, 48 hours) showed only 20% mortality.

- Flies exposed to PQ showed oxidative stress compared to the control group, whereas prophylaxis with BM averted the oxidative stress.
- Mitochondrial fractions obtained from the whole body homogenate of flies exposed to PQ showed decreased activities of electron transport chain (ETC) enzymes compared to the control group. Prophylaxis with BM for 7 days followed by PQ exposure prevented decreases in ETC enzyme activity.

Jadiya and coworkers[32] examined the effect of BM on Parkinson's disease using Caenorhabditis elegans. Two different strains of C. elegans were used: transgenic strain NL 5901 expressing human alpha synuclein protein; and transgenic strain BZ 555 expressing green fluorescent protein (GFP) specifically in the dopaminergic neurons. C. elegans contains two pairs of cephalic (CEP) neurons, one pair of anterior deirid (ADE) neurons in the head region, and a pair of posterior deirid (PDE) neurons in the posterior lateral region. Degeneration of these neurons was induced by 6-OHDA, a neurotoxin that has been reported to produce some of the behavioral, biochemical and pathological changes observed in Parkinson's disease. The results are summarized below:

- NL 5901 worms treated with BM showed a decrease in the aggregation of alpha synuclein compared to untreated NL 5901 worms.
- Untreated NL 5901 worms had less lipid content than normal (wild type) worms. NL 5901 worms treated with BM showed an increase in lipid content compared to untreated NL 5901 worms.
- BZ 555 worms treated with 6-OHDA showed diminution of GFP expression compared to untreated BZ 555 worms. BZ 555 worms treated with BM and exposed to 6-OHDA showed enhanced expression of GFP compared to BZ 555 worms exposed only to 6-OHDA, indicating protection of CEP, ADE and PDE neurons by BM.

The authors concluded that **"Bacopa monnieri reduces alpha synuclein aggregation, prevents dopaminergic neurodegeneration and restores the lipid content in nematodes, thereby proving its potential as a possible anti-parkinsonian agent."**

Nellore and coworkers[33] investigated the effect of platinum nanoparticles coated with Bacopa monniera (BME-PtNPs) on Parkinsonism in zebra fish induced by 1-methyl-4-phenyl-1,2,3,6-tetrahydro pyridine (MPTP).

MPTP is a neurotoxin and a precursor of 1-methyl-4-phenyl pyridinium (MPP+), which causes symptoms of PD in several species including zebra fish. The investigators used wild type adult zebra fish (under 8 months old) in their study. Zebra fish treated with MPTP (225 mg/kg, i.p) showed the following changes compared to the control group:

- Reduced locomotor activity
- Increased MDA levels and decreased GSH, SOD, CAT, GPx, DA, 3,4-dihydroxyphenylacetic acid and homovanilic acid (whole brain homogenate)
- Inhibited complex I activity (mitochondrial preparation)

Pretreatment with BME-PtNPs (0.4 μmol) reversed these changes. The authors attributed the neuroprotective effect of BME-PtNPs to their antioxidant activity as well as their ability to restore the activity of complex I in the mitochondrial respiratory chain.

Shobana and coworkers[34] examined the effect of an alcohol extract of Bacopa monniera (AEBM) on behavioral and biochemical changes induced by 6-OHDA in rats. Behavioral changes were evaluated by the locomotor, rotarod, grip, forced swim and radial arm maze tests. Male albino rats (5 months old) treated with ascorbic acid-saline for 21 days followed by 6-OHDA on day 22 showed the following changes compared to the control group:

- Behavioral impairment
- Increased LPO and decreased GSH (substantia nigra)
- Decreased GPx, GR, GST, SOD, CAT (striatum)

Rats treated with AEBM (20 or 40 mg/kg/day, PO) for 21 days followed by 6-OHDA on day 22 showed a reversal of these changes. The authors concluded that **"the extract of B. monniera might be helpful in attenuating 6-OHDA induced lesioning in rats."**

In a subsequent investigation, Shobana and Sumathi[35] evaluated the effect of bacoside A (BA) on behavioral and biochemical changes induced by 6-OHDA. The results of this study were largely similar to the previous one[34]. The authors concluded that **"bacoside A can be used as the best tool to prevent 6-hydroxy dopamine induced parkinsonism in rats."**

Swathi and coworkers[36] found that the administration of rotenone increased ACh and decreased AChE in various brain regions (cerebral cortex, cerebellum, midbrain, pons and medulla) of rats. Treatment with an alcohol extract of Bacopa monniera reversed these changes, comparable to the effect of L-dopa.

References

1 Parkinson's Disease Foundation. Statistics on Parkinson's. http://www.pdf.org/en/parkinson_statistics
2 Claudia Schulte, Thomas Gasser. Genetic basis of Parkinson's disease: inheritance, penetrance, and expression. The Application of Clinical Genetics (2011) 4: 67-80.
3 M C de Rijk, L J Launer, K Berger, M M Breteler, J F Dartigues, M Baldereschi, L Fratiglioni, A Lobo, J Martinez-Lage, C Trenkwalder, A Hofman. Prevalence of Parkinson's disease in Europe: a collaborative study of population-based cohorts. Neurologic diseases in the elderly research group. Neurology (2000) 54 (11 Suppl 5): S21-23.
4 Timothy J Collier, Nicholas M Kanaan, Jeffrey H Kordower. Aging as a primary risk factor for Parkinson's disease: evidence from studies of non-human primates. Nature Reviews Neuroscience (2011) 12: 359-366.
5 G F Wooten, L J Currie, V E Bovbjerg, J K Lee, J Patrie. Are men at greater risk for Parkinson's disease than women? Journal of Neurology, Neurosurgery & Psychiatry (2004) 75: 637–639.
6 Bobby Thomas, M Flint Beal. Molecular insights into Parkinson's disease. F-1000 Med Reports (2011). doi: 10. 3410/M3-7
7 Karen Nuytemans, Jessie Theuns, Marc Cruts, Christine Van Broeckhoven. Genetic etiology of Parkinson disease associated with mutations in the SNCA, PARK2, PINK1, PARK7 and LRRK2 genes: a mutation update. Human Mutation (2010) 31(7): 763-780.
8 Christine Klein, Ana Westenberger. Genetics of Parkinson's disease. Cold Spring Harb Perspect Med (2012) 2: a008888.
9 Yoshio Tsuboi. Environmental-genetic interactions in the pathogenesis of Parkinson's disease. Exp Neurobiology (2012) 21(3): 123-128.
10 Jill Stein, Ted Schettler, Ben Rohrer, Maria Valenti. "Environmental factors in the development of Parkinson's disease" in Environmental Threats to Healthy Aging with a Closer Look at Alzheimer's and Parkinson's Diseases. Edited by Nancy Myers. Greater Boston Physicians for Social Responsibility and Environmental Health Network, Boston, 2008.
11 A Priyadarshi, S A Khuder, E A Schaub, S S Priyadarshi. Environmental risk factors and Parkinson's disease: a metaanalysis. Environment Res (2001) 86(2): 122-127.
12 F D Dick, G De Palma, A Ahmadi, N W Scott, G J Prescott, J Bennett, S Semple, S Dick, C Counsell, P Mozzoni, N Haites, S Bezzina Wettinger, A Mutti, M Otelea, A Seaton, P Soderkvist, A Felice, on behalf of Geoparkinson study group. Environmental risk factors for Parkinson's disease and parkinsonism: the Geoparkinson study. Occup. Environ. Med. (2007) 64: 666-672.
13 R Kones. Parkinson's disease: mitochondrial molecular pathology, inflammation, statins and therapeutic neuroprotective nutrition. Nutr Clin Pract (2010) 25(4): 371-89.
14 Anthony H Schapira, Peter Jenner. Etiology and pathogenesis of Parkinson's disease. Movement Disorders (2011) 26(6): 1049-1055.

inflammation, statins and therapeutic neuroprotective nutrition. Nutr Clin Pract (2010) 25(4): 371-89.

14 Anthony H Schapira, Peter Jenner. Etiology and pathogenesis of Parkinson's disease. Movement Disorders (2011) 26(6): 1049-1055.

15 Kim Tieu. A guide to neurotoxic animal models of Parkinson's disease. Cold Spring Harp Perspect Med 2011: doi: 10.1101/cshperspect.a009316.

16 V Munoz-Soriano, N Paricio. Drosophila models of Parkinson's disease: discovering relevant pathways and novel therapeutic strategies. Parkinson's Disease (2011). Article ID 520640, 14 pages. doi: 10.4061/2011/520640

17 S Mullin, A Schapira. α-Synuclein and mitochondrial dysfunction in Parkinson's disease. Molecular Neurobiology (2013) 47: 587-597.

18 John G Nutt, G Frederick Wooten. Diagnosis and initial management of Parkinson's disease. N Engl J Med (2005) 353(10): 1021-1027.

19 Joao Massano, Kailash P Bhatia. Clinical approach to Parkinson's disease: features, diagnosis and principles of management. Cold Spring Harb Perspect Med (2012). doi: 10.1101/cshperspect.a00870

20 Sherri Damlo. AAN releases recommendation on treatment of Parkinson's disease. American Family physician (2007) 75(6): 922-924.

21 Daniel Tarsy. Patient information: Parkinson disease treatment options – medications (beyond the basics). Section Editor. Howard I Hurtig. Deputy Editor. John F Dashe. http://www.uptodate.com/contents/parkinson-disease-treatment-options-medications-beyond-the-basics

22 M Gourie-Devi, M G Ramu, B S Venkataram. Treatment of Parkinson's disease in 'Ayurveda' (ancient Indian system of medicine): discussion paper. Journal of the Royal Society of Medicine (1991) 84: 491-492.

23 Lakshmi Chandra Mishra, R H Singh." Parkinson's disease (kampa vata)" in Scientific Basis for Ayurvedic Therapies. Edited by Lakshmi Chandra Mishra. CRC Press, Boca Raton, FL 2004.

24 Nayak Annada Prasad. Parkinsonism in Ayurvedic perspective, a bird's eye view. Global J. Res. Med. Plants & Indigen. Med. (2012) 1(11): 629-638.

25 C Andrade, T Raj, H B Udaya, S Chandra. Effect of BR-16A on alpha-2 adrenergic, dopamine autoreceptor and dopamine postsynaptic receptor functioning. Indian Journal of Pharmacology (1994) 26: 292-295.

26 C Andrade. The herbal treatment of Parkinson's disease: a possible role for BR-16A (Mentat). Ind. J. Psychol. Med. (1996) 19(2): 82.

27 Ravikumar Hosamani, Muralidhara. Neuroprotective efficacy of Bacopa monnieri against rotenone induced oxidative stress and neurotoxicity in drosophila melanogaster. NeuroToxicology (2009) 30: 977-985.

28 George K Shinomol, Rajeswara Babu Mythri, M M Srinivas Bharath, Muralidhara. Bacopa monnieri extract offsets rotenone-induced cytotoxicity in dopaminergic cells and oxidative impairments in mice brain. Cell Mol Neurobiol (2012) 32: 455-465.

29 Gunduluru Swathi, Gopalreddygari Visweswari, Wudayagiri Rajendra. Evaluation of rotenone induced Parkinson's disease on glutamate metabolism and protective strategies of Bacopa monnieri. International Journal of Plant, Animal and Environmental Sciences (2013) 3(1): 62-67.

30 Gunduluru Swathi, Cherukupalle Bhuvaneswar, Wudayagiri Rajendra.

monnieri leaf powder mitigates paraquat-induced oxidative perturbations and lethality in drosophila melanogaster. Indian Journal of Biochemistry and Biophysics (2010) 47: 75-82.

32 Pooja Jadiya, Asif Khan, Shreesh Raj Sammi, Supinder Kaur, Snober S Mir, Aamir Nazir. Anti-parkinsonian effects of Bacopa monnieri; insights from transgenic and pharmacological Caenorhabditis elegans models of Parkinson's disease. Biochemical and Biophysical Research Communications (2011) 413(4): 605-610.

33 Jayashree Nellore, Cynthia Pauline, Kanchana Amarnath. Bacopa monnieri phytochemicals mediated synthesis of platinum nanoparticles and its neurorescue effect on 1-methyl 4-phenyl 1,2,3,6 tetrahydropyridine-induced experimental parkinsonism in zebrafish. Journal of Neurodegenerative Diseases (2013). doi: 10.1155/2013/972391

34 Chandrasekar Shobana, Radhakrishnan Ramesh Kumar, Thangarajan Sumathi. Alcoholic extract of Bacopa monniera linn. protects against 6-hydroxydopamine-induced changes in behavioral and biochemical aspects: a pilot study. Cell Mol Neurobiol (2012) 32: 1099-1112.

35 Chandrasekar Shobana, Thangarajan Sumathi. Studies on behavioral, biochemical, immunohistochemical and quantification of dopamine and its metabolites in the striatum of 6-hydroxy dopamine induced parkinsonism in rats – attenuation by bacoside-A, a major phytoconstituent of Bacopa monniera. IJABPT (2013) 4(4): 120-142.

36 Gunduluru Swathi, Cherukupalle Bhuvaneswar, Wudayagiri Rajendra. Alterations of cholinergic neurotransmission in rotenone induced Parkinson's disease: protective role of Bacopa monnieri. International Journal of Pharmacy and Biological Sciences (2013) 3(2): 286-292.

8 – Anxiolytic and Antidepressant Activity

8.1 – General

Anxiety is an emotion that everyone experiences from time to time. It is generally a feeling of apprehension, fear, and worry. Some degree of anxiety may be beneficial if it can prepare one to face stressful situations. If symptoms are severe, occur for no apparent reason, and continue for a long time, they are harmful and viewed as an anxiety disorder[1]. The term anxiety disorder refers to a heterogeneous group of disorders, each of which has its own symptoms. The exact causes of most anxiety disorders are unknown, but they probably stem from biological, psychological, and sociological factors. Anxiety disorders are widespread in the general population. In the US, about 40 million adults (age 18 and older) are affected in a given year[2]. In surveys conducted across a number of western countries, lifetime prevalence rates range from 13.6% to 28.8%[3].

Depression is another common mental disorder. Most people experience feelings like sadness, helplessness and frustration for short periods of time. However, if the symptoms persist for longer periods and impair daily activities, they are harmful and referred to as depression. Symptoms of depression include sadness, loss of pleasure, inability to concentrate, fatigue, irregular sleep or appetite, feelings of worthlessness or guilt, and thoughts of suicide[1,4]. As with anxiety, depression is a heterogeneous group of disorders. Its exact cause is unknown, and it is a serious health issue all over the world. In the US, an estimated one in ten adults suffers from depression[5]. Globally, depression is the leading cause of disability, with more than 350 million people affected[6].

Anxiety and depression may occur together. If untreated, either or both can cause severe distress, difficulty with work, difficulty with forming and maintaining social relationships, and an overall deterioration in the quality of life. Although conventional treatments are fairly effective, they can also cause undesirable side effects and are often expensive. For these reasons and others, a large number of people affected by these disorders do not seek conventional treatments. Many seek out complementary and alternative medicine (CAM) therapies instead. In 1997-8, a survey of 2055 people showed that 57% of those suffering from anxiety attacks and 54% suffering from depression used CAM therapies[7].

8.2 – Ayurveda and Anxiety and Depression

The Ayurvedic concept of mental disorders includes cittodvega (anxiety) and cittavasada (depression)[8]. In the Ayurvedic model, impairment of the rajas and tamas gunas (mentioned earlier in section 1.2.2) causes anger, greed, lust, delusion, envy, pride, euphoria, grief and anxiety[9]. Ayurveda utilizes three main approaches for the management of mental disorders[10]:

- Daiva Vyapashraya – Spiritual therapy that includes the use of mantra, japa (meditation), and other religious activities.
- Satvavajaya – Psychotherapy
- Yukti Vypashraya – Biological therapy that includes cleansing followed by palliative treatment with herbal drugs, dietetics, and lifestyle improvements. Single herbs as well as polyherbal formulations are used, with most of the herbal drugs belonging to the medhya rasayana category. Research on medicinal plants with anxiolytic and antidepressant potential has considerably increased during the last few decades[11-19].

8.3 – Animal Studies

Bhattacharya and Ghosal[20] investigated the anxiolytic activity of an ethanol extract of Bacopa monniera (BM) in rats. The anxiolytic activity of BM was compared to lorazepam, a standard antianxiety drug belonging to the benzodiazepine family. Charles Foster (CF) strain male rats were treated with the vehicle, BM (5, 10 or 20 mg/kg, PO), or lorazepam (0.5 mg/kg, i.p.). The rats were subjected to the open field, elevated plus maze, social interaction, and novelty suppressed feeding latency tests. All tests indicated anxiolytic activity of BM. The effect of BM at higher doses was greater than lorezapam. BM has an advantage over lorazepam because it is known to enhance cognition, whereas lorazepam induces amnesia.

Sairam and coworkers[21] evaluated the antidepressant activity of a methanol extract of Bacopa monniera (BME) in rats. CF albino rats were treated with the vehicle, BME (20 or 40 mg/kg/day, PO), or imipramine (15 mg/kg/day, i.p.) for 5 days. Imipramine is a standard antidepressant. The animals from each group were subjected to the forced swim and learned helplessness tests on day 6. Both tests indicated anxiolytic activity of BM. At higher doses, BM was more effective than imipramine.

Zhou and coworkers[22] isolated bacopaside I, bacopaside II, bacopaside VII and bacopasaponin C from Bacopa monniera and examined their antidepressant activity in mice. Mice treated with these compounds (50 mg/kg/day, PO, 7 days) were subjected to the forced swim and tail suspension tests. Fluoxetine (10 mg/kg/day, PO, 7 days) was also examined. Both tests indicated anxiolytic activity of bacopaside I, bacopaside II and bacopasaponin C. The effect decreased in the order bacopaside I > bacopasaponin C > bacopaside II. The effect of bacopaside I was comparable to fluoxetine. Bacopaside I, bacopaside II and bacopasaponin C have the same aglycone, whereas bacopaside VII has a different aglycone. The authors observed that **"it seems that the aglycone plays the crucial role for the antidepressant activity of these compounds."**

Chatterji and coworkers[23] evaluated the effect of an ethanol extract of Bacopa monniera (BM) on mixed anxiety-depressive disorder in mice. The results were compared with ginseng, diazepam, and imipramine. Anxiety was evaluated by the light-dark, elevated plus maze and hole-board tests. The light-dark and elevated plus maze tests indicated anxiolytic activity of BM. Ginseng and diazepam showed a greater effect. The hole-board test indicated anxiolytic activity of ginseng and diazepam, but not BM. The authors suggested that Bacopa monniera has a different mechanism of anxiolytic action than ginseng or diazepam.

Depression was evaluated by the tail suspension and forced swim tests. In the tail suspension test, BM and ginseng showed comparable antidepressant activity. Imipramine showed a greater effect. The forced swim test indicated antidepressant activity of BM. Ginseng and imipramine showed a greater effect.

Maity and coworkers[24] conducted a comparative study of the antidepressant effect of Bacopa monniera (BM), Withania somnifera (WS), Imipramine (IMP), BM+IMP and WS+IMP in rats. These agents were administered for 14 days. Antidepressant activity was evaluated by the forced swim and learned helplessness tests. The results are summarized below:

- In the forced swim test, antidepressant activity decreased in the following order: IMP (16 mg) + WS (50 mg) > WS (150 mg) > IMP (64 mg) > IMP (16 mg) + BM (20 mg) > BM (80 mg).
- In the learned helplessness test, antidepressant activity decreased in the following order: IMP (16 mg) + WS (50 mg) > IMP (64 mg) > WS (150 mg) > IMP (16 mg) + BM (20 mg) > BM (80 mg).

The BM group did not exhibit significant antidepressant activity at low doses. However, BM was effective even at low doses when given along with low doses of IMP.

Abbas and coworkers[25] investigated the antidepressant effect of a hydro ethanolic extract (HE-ext) and an n-butanol extract (n-Bt-ext) of Bacopa monniera in mice using the forced swim, tail suspension and yohimbine toxicity tests. The results are summarized below:

- In the forced swim test, both HE-ext (40-160 mg/kg, i.p.) and n-Bt-ext (80 mg/kg, i.p.) showed antidepressant activity. The effect produced by HE-ext (80 mg) or n-Bt-ext (80 mg) was comparable to fluoxetine (45 mg/kg, i.p.).
- In the tail suspension test, n-Bt-Ext (80 mg/kg, i.p.) showed antidepressant activity comparable to fluoxetine (45 mg/kg, i.p.), whereas HE-ext (40-160 mg/kg, i.p.) did not show a significant effect.
- The yohimbine toxicity test was conducted by treating mice with saline (control), HE-ext (40-80 mg/kg), n-Bt-ext (80 mg/kg) or imipramine (20-80 mg/kg). After an hour, yohimbine (30 mg/kg, SC) was administered. Both n-Bt-ext and imipramine (40 or 80 mg) potentiated yohimbine-induced mortality to 75% compared to the control group, whereas HE-ext did not, indicating the possibility of the involvement of biogenic amines for the antidepressant effect of n-Bt-ext.

Mishra and coworkers[26] assessed the antidepressant activity of anximin in CF albino rats. Anximin is a polyherbal formulation that contains Bacopa monniera. Rats were treated with either the vehicle (control), anximin (20 or 40 mg/kg/day, PO) or imipramine (10 mg/kg/day, PO) for 7 days. The rats were subjected to the forced swim, tail suspension, learned helplessness and yohimbine toxicity tests. The results are summarized below:

- In the forced swim, tail suspension, and learned helplessness tests, anximin showed antidepressant activity. The effect of anximin (40 mg/kg) was comparable to imipramine.
- At 20 and 40 mg doses of anximin, yohimbine administration caused 33% and 66% lethality, respectively. Imipramine followed by yohimbine administration resulted in 100% mortality.

A receptor binding study was done to elucidate the mechanism of antidepressant action. The results suggested the involvement of the 5-HT_{2A} receptor in antidepressant activity.

Hazra and coworkers[27] studied the antidepressant activity of a Bacopa monniera extract using the stress-induced animal model of depression. Stress was induced by foot shocks. Rats treated with the vehicle and given foot shocks for 21 days followed by foot shocks on alternate days for the next 9 days showed progressive loss of weight, depressive behavior and increased plasma corticosterone compared to the control group. Rats treated with the vehicle and given foot shocks for 21 days followed by treatment with Bacopa monniera extract (40, 80, or 120 mg/kg/day, PO) or fluoxetine (10 mg/kg/day, i.p.) for the next 7 days showed a reversal of these changes.

8.4 – Clinical Trials

Singh and coworkers[28] evaluated the anxiolytic activity of Bacopa monniera in human subjects. In an open trial, 35 subjects diagnosed with anxiety disorder were treated with a 30 mL syrup of Bacopa monniera (equivalent to 12 g of crude drug) per day in two equal doses for four weeks. The subjects were evaluated for anxiety level, maladjustment, mental fatigue rate, immediate memory span, disability level, and physical and chemical status before commencement (baseline) and after completion of the treatment. The following improvements were noted after the treatment:

- Reduction in anxiety level
- Reduced maladjustment rate, disability level and mental fatigue rate
- Improved immediate memory span
- Slight reduction in average systolic pressure
- Significant improvement in respiratory function
- Reduced levels of urinary vanillylmandelic acid and corticosteroid excretion

Also, the subjects reported relief from other symptoms of anxiety such as insomnia, headache, irritability, lack of concentration, anorexia, dyspepsia, tremors, palpitations and nervousness.

In an open trial, Yadav and coworkers[29] studied the effect of Bacopa monniera on normal subjects (n=16) and those diagnosed with anxiety disorder (n=18). The subjects were treated with Bacopa monniera capsules (equivalent to 2.5 g of dry herb) three times daily for four weeks. Subjects showed improvements in anxiety level, depression level, mental fatigue, memory span and systolic blood pressure. Reductions in nervousness, palpitations, headaches and insomnia were also reported. The effects were more significant in subjects with anxiety disorder than in normal subjects.

In a double-blind, placebo-controlled trial, Stough and coworkers[30] randomly assigned 46 healthy volunteers (18-60 years old) to either a Bacopa monniera group or a placebo group. Subjects in the Bacopa monniera group were treated with a Bacopa monniera extract daily for 12 weeks. After the treatment, subjects in the Bacopa monniera group showed a decrease in anxiety compared to the placebo group. Another double-blind, placebo-controlled trial[31] in which 54 healthy volunteers (age 65 or older) participated over a period of 12 weeks showed a decrease in anxiety and depression after treatment with a Bacopa monniera (300 mg/day) extract.

Roodenrys and coworkers[32] conducted a double-blind, placebo-controlled trial in which 84 healthy volunteers (40-65 years old) were randomly assigned to either a Bacopa monniera or a placebo group. Subjects in the Bacopa monniera group were treated with a Bacopa monniera extract (450 mg/day for subjects over 90 kg body weight and 300 mg/day for subjects under 90 kg) daily for three months. After the treatment period, no significant improvements in subjective measures of psychological state (depression, anxiety and stress) were observed compared to the placebo group.

Bhargava and Khan[33] evaluated the efficacy and side effects of imipramine, sertraline and an Ayurvedic formulation in clinically depressed patients. Imipramine belongs to the tricyclic antidepressant group and sertraline to the selective serotonin reuptake inhibitor group. The Ayurvedic formulation contained Bacopa monniera and other herbs. 90 subjects diagnosed with depression (18-60 years old) participated in the study. They were divided into three main groups and treated for 12 weeks as follows:

Group	Treatment
1	Imipramine (75-150 mg/day), once daily
2	Sertraline (50-150 mg/day), once daily
3	Ayurvedic formulation (1000 mg/day), in the dose of 500 mg twice daily

The imipramine group showed progressive declines in depression scores from the 4th week to the 12th week, whereas the sertraline and Ayurvedic formulation groups showed progressive declines in depression scores from the 2nd week to the 12th week. At the end of the 12th week, the Ayurvedic formulation produced the best results overall. The side effects are summarized below in decreasing order of incidence:

- Imipramine – Sedation, dry mouth, tachycardia, abdominal discomfort, tremors, sexual dysfunction, weight gain, urinary retention and agitation
- Sertraline – Nausea, abdominal discomfort, dry mouth, weight gain, sexual dysfunction and tachycardia
- Ayurvedic formulation – Negligible

References

1 DSM-IV-TR: Diagnostic and statistical manual of mental disorders, fourth edition, text revision. American Psychiatric Association, Arlington, VA, 2000.
2 Ronald C Kessler, Wai Tat Chiu, Olga Demler, Ellen E Walters. Prevalence, severity, and comorbidity of 12-month old DSM-IV disorders in the national comorbidity survey replication. Arch Gen Psychiatry (2005) 62: 617-627.
3 Tanja Michael, Ulrike Zetsche, Jurgen Margraf. Epidemiology of anxiety disorders. Psychiatry (2007) 6(4): 136-142.
4 C H Duman. “Models of depression: in Vitamins and Hormones; Hormones of the Limbic system Vol 82. Edited by Gerald Litwack. Academic Press, 2010.
5 Centers for Disease Control and Prevention. An Estimated 1 in 10 U.S. Adults Report Depression. Atlanta, GA, 2011. http://www.cdc.gov/features/dsdepression/
6 World Health Organization. Depression: fact sheet no. 369. October 2012.
7 Ronald C Kessler, Jane Soukup, Roger B Davis, David F Foster, Sonja A Wilkey, Maria I Van Rompay, David M Eisenberg. The use of complementary and alternative therapies to treat anxiety and depression in the United States. Am J Psychiatry (2001) 158(2): 289-294.
8 Hemant K Singh. Brain enhancing ingredients from Ayurvedic medicine: quintessential example of Bacopa monniera, a narrative review. Nutrients (2013) 5: 478-497.
9 R K Sharma and Bhagwan Dash. Caraka Samhita (text with English translation and critical exposition based on Cakrapani Datta’s Ayurveda Dipika) volume 2. Chowkhamba Sanskrit Series Office, Varanasi, India, Reprint 2007.
10 R H Singh, Lakshmi Chandra Mishra. “Psychiatric Disorders” in Scientific Basis for Ayurvedic Therapies. Edited by Lakshmi Chandra Mishra. CRC press, Boca Raton, FL 2004.
11 Jerome Sarris, Alexander Panossian, Isaac Schweitzer, Con Stough, Andrew Scholey. Herbal medicine for depression, anxiety and insomnia: a review of psychopharmacology and clinical evidence. European Neuropsychopharmacology (2011) 21: 841-860.
12 M Sharma, S Sahu, N Khemani, R Kaur. Ayurvedic medicinal plants as psychotherapeutic agents – a review. International Journal of Applied Biology and Pharmaceutical Technology (2013) 4(2): 214-218.
13 B V Rao, B N Srikumar, B S S Rao. “Herbal remedies to treat anxiety

disorders" in Different Views of Anxiety Disorders. Edited by S Selek. InTech (2011). doi: 10.5772/23511

14 Madhuri D Bhujbal, Poonam Bangar, Dhanaji D Ghanwat. A review of medicinal plant exhibiting anxiolytic activity. International Journal of Universal Pharmacy and Bio Sciences (2012) 1(1): 26-38.

15 Priyanka Thakur, A C Rana. Anxiolytic potential of medicinal plants. IJNPND (2013) 3(4): 325-331.

16 Dinesh Dhingra, Amandeep Sharma. A review on antidepressant plants. Natural Product Radiance (2006) 5(2): 144 – 152.

17 Mithun Singh Rajput, Sampada Sinha, Vineet Mathur, Purti Agrawal. Herbal antidepressants. IJPFR (2011) 1(1): 159-169.

18 Talha Jawaid, Roli Gupta, Zohaib Ahmed Siddiqui. A review on herbal plants showing antidepressant activity. International Journal of Pharmaceutical Sciences and Research (2011) 2(12): 3051-3060.

19 Rupesh K Gautam, Praveen K Dixit, Suchita Mittal. Herbal sources of antidepressant potential: a review. International Journal of Pharmaceutical Sciences Review and Research (2013) 18(1): 86-91.

20 S K Bhattacharya, S Ghosal. Anxiolytic activity of a standardized extract of Bacopa monniera: an experimental study. Phytomedicine (1998) 5(2): 77-82.

21 K Sairam, M Dorababu, R K Goel, S K Bhattacharya. Antidepressant activity of standardized extract of Bacopa monniera in experimental models of depression in rats. Phytomedicine (2002) 9: 207-211.

22 Yun Zhou, Yun-Heng Shen, Chuan Zhang, Juan Su, Run-Hui Liu, Wei-Dong Zhang. Triterpene saponins from Bacopa monnieri and their antidepressant effects in two mice models. J. Nat. Prod. (2007) 70: 652-655.

23 M Chatterjee, P Verma, G Palit. Comparative evaluation of Bacopa monniera and Panax quniquefolium in experimental anxiety and depressive models in mice. Indian Journal of Experimental Biology (2010) 48: 306-313.

24 T Maity, A Adhikari, K Bhattacharya, S Biswas, P K Debnath, C S Maharana. A study on evaluation of antidepressant effect of imipramine adjunct with aswagandha and Brahmi. Nepal Med Coll J (2011) 13(4): 250-253.

25 Muzaffar Abbas, Fazal Subhan, Khalid Rauf, Munasib Khan, Syed Nadeem-ul-Hassan Mohani. The involvement of biogenic amines in the antidepressant effect of Bacopa monnieri. Pharmacologyonline (2011) 1: 112-123.

26 S Mishra, V K Khanna, Vikas Kumar. 5-HT_{2A} receptor binding and antidepressant studies on Anximin, a polyherbal formulation. Pharmacologyonline (2008) 2: 379-389.

27 Somoday Hazra, Ritabrata Banerjee, Biplab K Das, Anup K Ghosh, Tarit K Banerjee, Uday S Hazra, Susanta K Biswas, Amal C Mondal. Evaluation of antidepressant activity of Bacopa monnieri in rat: a study in animal model of depression. Drug discovery (2012) 2(4): 8-13.

28 R H Singh, L Singh. Studies on the anti-anxiety effect of the medhya rasayana drug, Brahmi (Bacopa monniera wettst), part I. J Res Ayur Siddha (1981) 1(1): 133-148.

29 R K Yadav, R H Singh. A clinical and experimental study on medhya effect of Aindri (Bacopa monnieri Linn). J Res Ayur Siddha (1996) 17(1-2): 1-15.

30 C Stough, J Lloyd, J Clarke, L A Downey, C W Hutchison, T Rodgers, P J Nathan. The chronic effects of an extract of Bacopa monniera (Brahmi) on cognitive function in healthy human subjects. Psychopharmacology (2001) 156: 481-484.

31 Carlo Calabrese, William L Gregory, Micheal Leo, Dale Kraemer, Kerry Bone, Barry Oken. Effects of a standardized Bacopa monnieri extract on cognitive performance, anxiety and depression in the elderly: a randomized double-blind, placebo-controlled trial. J. Altern. Comp. Med. (2008) 14(6): 707-713.

32 Steven Roodenrys, Dianne Booth, Sonia Bulzomi, Andrew Phipps, Caroline Micallef, Jaclyn Smoker. Chronic effects of Brahmi (Bacopa monnieri) on human memory. Neuropsychopharmacology (2002) 27(2): 279-281.

33 J Bhargava, Z Y Khan. Comparative evaluation of the efficacy and side effects of imipramine, sertraline and an Ayurvedic formulation in patients of depression. Journal of Clinical and Diagnostic Research (2012) 6(2): 220-225.

9 – Effect on ADHD and ASD

9.1 – Attention Deficit Hyperactivity Disorder

9.1.1 – General

Attention deficit hyperactivity disorder (ADHD) is a chronic neurobehavioral disorder of childhood that often continues into adolescence and adulthood. The pooled worldwide prevalence of ADHD has been estimated to be 5.29% in children and adolescents, and 2.5-4.4% among adults[1,2]. Primary characteristics of ADHD include inattention, impulsiveness and hyperactivity[3]. ADHD may cause serious impairments in academic, social and interpersonal functioning[4].

The exact causes of ADHD are still unknown. Both genetic and environmental factors are considered to play a role in the development of the disorder[6]. Imaging studies have shown an overall reduction in brain size associated with ADHD[7]. Neuropharmacological studies have indicated dysregulation of both noradrenaline and dopamine neurotransmitter systems[8].

There is no specific laboratory test for ADHD. The diagnosis is based on the observation of certain behavioral symptoms. The American Psychiatric Association's Diagnostic and Statistical Manual IV, text revision (DSM-IV-TR) is used by mental health professionals to help diagnose ADHD[5].

At present there is no cure for ADHD, but treatments are available to successfully manage the symptoms. The treatment includes medication, counseling and cognitive behavioral therapies. Medication is the mainstay of the treatment and stimulants like methylphenidate and amphetamine compounds are the most commonly prescribed drugs. Nonstimulants, atypical antidepressants and certain blood pressure medications are also used in the treatment of ADHD[9].

9.1.2 – Ayurveda and ADHD

ADHD has not been described as a specific disease in Ayurveda, but based on the symptoms, it is likely due to vata or vata/pitta imbalances[10]. Treatment is given to correct the imbalance, taking into consideration the unique prakriti of the individual. Therapies include lifestyle changes such as steady routines, proper diet, avoidance of excessive stimulation, herbal medicines, yoga and meditation. Among the herbs, Brahmi has become popular in the treatment of ADHD. Its efficacy has been evaluated in a number of scientific investigations.

9.1.3 – Experimental Evidence

Negi and coworkers[11] conducted a double-blind, randomized, placebo-controlled study to evaluate the efficacy of Bacopa monniera in the treatment of children with ADHD. Thirty six school age children diagnosed with ADHD were assigned to either a Bacopa group (n=19, mean age=8.3) or placebo group (n=17, mean age=9.3). The children in the Bacopa group received 50 mg of Bacopa monniera extract twice daily for 12 weeks. Children in the Bacopa group performed better than the placebo group in the areas of sentence repetition, logical memory and paired associative learning after 12 weeks of treatment. At the 16th week, these improvements were maintained even after terminating Bacopa monniera treatment four weeks earlier.

The efficacy of Mentat (a proprietary preparation of Bacopa monniera) has been evaluated in the treatment of ADHD by a number of investigators[12-14]. Kalra and coworkers[14] conducted a double-blind, placebo-controlled clinical trial with 60 ADHD children. They were divided into two groups. One group (n=30) received Mentat and the other received a placebo for six months. Assessment of academic functioning and psychological tests were done before and after the treatment. Children treated with Mentat showed improvements in ADHD symptoms.

Singhal and coworkers[15] examined the effect of a polyherbal formulation containing Bacopa monniera (PHF), both by itself and in combination with Shirodhara therapy, on reaction time in ADHD children. (Children with ADHD have slower reaction times than the general population). Shirodhara was performed by pouring milk over the forehead of the subject from a height of 3.14 inches for 45 min/day for two weeks. Children (6 to 16 years old) diagnosed with ADHD were randomly assigned to one of three groups and treated as follows:

- Group A (n=17): PHF syrup (1.0 mL/kg/day) in three equal doses for three months

- Group B (n=14): PHF syrup (1.0 mL/kg/day) in three equal doses for three months and shirodhara for two weeks
- Group C (n=12): Placebo syrup

Reaction times were measured before and after the treatment. After the treatment, groups A and B showed decreases in both visual and auditory reaction times compared to the corresponding initial values, whereas group C did not show a significant decrease. Both groups A and B showed decreases in overall reaction time, with group B showing a greater effect.

Katz and coworkers[16] conducted a double-blind, randomized, placebo-controlled trial to examine the efficacy of a compound herbal preparation (CHP) in the treatment of children with ADHD. The CHP contained Bacopa monniera and other herbs. Children diagnosed with ADHD (6-12 years old) were randomly assigned to either a treatment group (n=80) or a control group (n=40). Participants were accordingly treated with CHP or a placebo over a four month period. The participants were administered the test of variables of attention (TOVA) before the start and after the end of the treatment period. TOVA is a widely used computerized test of attention and impulsivity. 91% of participants in the treatment group completed the study, along with 48% from the control group. The treatment group showed improvements in all four subscales of TOVA as well as in overall TOVA scores. The control group showed no improvements.

9.2 – Autism Spectrum Disorders

9.2.1 – General

Autism spectrum disorders (ASD, or Autism) represent a group of neurodevelopmental disorders. Core symptoms include impairments in social interaction and communication, repetitive or stereotypic behavior and a restricted narrow range of interests. The symptoms appear in the first three years of life[17]. The global prevalence of autism has been estimated to be 62 out of 10,000 people[18], and boys are five times more likely to develop autism than girls[19]. The exact causes of ASD are not known. Both genetic and non-genetic factors[20-22] have been found to increase susceptibility to ASD.

ASD is diagnosed according to guidelines listed in the DSM-IV-TR[5]. The manual specifies five disorders, called pervasive developmental disorders (PDDs), as belonging to ASD: Autistic disorder (classic autism), Asperger's disorder (Asperger's syndrome), pervasive developmental disorder not otherwise specified (PDD-NOS), Rett disorder (Rett syndrome) and childhood disintegrative disorder (Heller's syndrome).

There is currently no cure for ASD. However, a variety of therapies are available[23] to manage the symptoms: applied behavioral analysis, medications, and occupational, physical, speech and language therapy. Intervention strategies should be selected to suit the individual's needs as early as possible. Medicines are used to treat the comorbid symptoms of ASD that often include seizures, sleep problems, gastrointestinal disorders, anxiety, ADHD and depression.

9.2.2 – Ayurveda and ASD

The symptoms of ASD are described under the category of unmada in Ayurveda. The Charaka Samhita states[24]:

> unmadam punarmanobudhi samjnajnanam smriti bhakti
> sheela chesta achara vighram vidyat unmada

Unmada is characterized by disturbed conditions of Manas (mind), Budhi (intellect), Samjnajnanam (consciousness), Smriti (memory), Bhakti (desire), Sheela (manners), Chesta (activities), and Achara (habits).

The cause of autism from the Ayurvedic perspective has been explained recently by Yadav and coworkers[25]. Impairments of pranavayu, udanavayu and vyanavayu have been suggested. These support the mind, heart, sense organs, intelligence, inspiration, initiation of speech and a number of other functions[26]. Ramachandran and Ramya[27] have recently described some interventions for childhood autism with certain Ayurvedic drugs and procedures. In the Ayurvedic treatment of ASD, diet plays an important role. The children should be given sattvic food that pacifies vata. A number of Ayurvedic treatments for ASD have been reported in the literature and are listed below[25,28,29]:

- Medhya rasayanas to improve mental functions, and other herbal medicines to improve digestive functions
- Massage with medicated oils
- Shirodhara
- Emesis and purgation
- Enema
- Nasya

9.2.3 – Experimental Evidence

Sandhya and coworkers[30] showed that an aqueous extract of Bacopa monniera (BM) ameliorated behavioral alterations and decreased oxidative stress markers in autistic rats. Rats on gestation for 12.5 days were divided into two groups. One group was given sodium valproate (VPA, 600 mg/kg, i.p.) and the other was given saline (control). The pups of rats treated with sodium valproate showed autistic symptoms. After weaning (PND-20), male pups were divided into three groups and treated as follows:

- Group 1 – Normal pups were treated with saline from PND-21 to PND-35 (control group)
- Group 2 – Autistic pups were treated with saline from PND-21 to PND-35
- Group 3 – Autistic pups were treated with BM (300 mg/kg/day, PO) from PND-21 to PND-35

From PND-30 to PND-40 (adolescent period) and PND-90 to PND-110 (adulthood period), the pups were subjected to a number of behavioral tests. The pups were sacrificed on PND-110. The results are summarized below (Table 9.1):

Test/Assay	Autistic pups (2) compared to Control (1)	Autistic pups + BM (3) compared to Autistic pups (2)
Pain sensitivity, exploratory and social activities	Decreased	Increased
Locomotor activity and anxiety	Increased	Decreased
5-HT, total nitrite (hippocampus)	Increased	Decreased
GSH, CAT (hippocampus)	Decreased	Increased

Table 9.1: Effects of BM on behavior alteration, oxidative stress and histoarchitecture in autistic rats

The authors concluded that an **"aqueous extract of Bacopa monniera may be beneficial in the treatment of autism."**

References

1 Guilherme Polanczyk, Luis Augusto Rohde. Epidemiology of attention-deficit/hyperactivity disorder across the lifespan. Current opinion in psychiatry (2007) 20(4): 386-392.

2 V Simon, P Czobor, S Balint, A Mesazaros, I Bitter. Prevalence and correlates of adult attention-deficit hyperactivity disorder: meta-analysis. Br J Psychiatry (2009) 194(3): 204-211.

3 R A Barkley. Attention-Deficit Hyperactivity Disorder, Third Edition: A Handbook for Diagnosis and Treatment. The Guilford Press, New York, 2005.

4 V A Harpin. The effect of ADHD on the life of an individual, their family, and community from preschool to adult life. Arch Dis Child (2005). doi: 10.1136/adc.2004.059006

5 DSM-IV-TR: Diagnostic and statistical manual of mental disorders, fourth edition, text revision. American Psychiatric Association, Arlington, VA, 2000.

6 Barry W Row, David Gozal. "Intermittent hypoxia during sleep as a model of environmental (nongenetic) contributions to attention deficit hyperactivity disorder" in Attention Deficit Hyperactivity Disorder From Genes to Patients. Edited by D Gozal, D L Molfese. Humana Press, Totowa, NJ, 2005.

7 Gail Tripp, Jeffery R Wickens. Neurobiology of ADHD. Neuropharmacology (2009) 57: 579-589.

8 Paolo Curatolo, Elisa D'Agati, Romina Moavero. The neurobiological basis of ADHD. Italian Journal of Pediatrics (2010) 36: 79.

9 Edward M Hallowell, John J Ratey. Delivered from distraction. Ballantine Books, New York, 2005.

10 Ann McIntyre. Herbal Treatment of Children: Western and Ayurvedic Perspectives. Elsevier Health Sciences, 2005.

11 K S Negi, Y D Singh, K P Kushwaha, C K Rastogi, A K Rathi, J S Srivastava, O P Asthana, R C Gupta, G Lucknow. Clinical evaluation of memory enhancing properties of Memory Plus in children with attention deficit hyperactivity disorder. Indian Journal of Psychiatry (2000) 42: supplement.

12 Bernard D D'souza, K B Chavda: Mentat in hyperactivity and attention deficiency disorders: a double-blind, placebo-controlled study. Probe (1991) 3(30): 227-232.

13 R B Patel, L P Pereira. Experience with Mentat in hyperkinetic children. Probe (1991) 30(3): 271-274.

14 Veena Kalra, Hina Zamir, R M Pandey, Kala Suhas Kulkarni. A randomized double blind placebo-controlled drug trial with Mentat in children with attention deficit hyperactivity disorder. Neurosciences Today (2002) 6(4): 223-227.

15 Harish Kumar Singhal, Neetu, Abhimanyu Kumar, Moti Rai. Ayurvedic approach for improving reaction time of attention deficit hyperactivity disorder affected children. Ayu (2010) 31(3): 338-342.

16 M Katz, A Adar Levine, H Kol-Degani, L Kav-Venaki. A compound herbal preparation (CHP) in the treatment of children with ADHD: a randomized

controlled trial. Journal of Attention Disorders (2010) 14(3): 281-291.

17 The National Institute of Mental Health. A Parent's Guide to Autism Spectrum Disorder. U.S Department of Health and Human Services (2011). NIH Publication No. 11-5511.

18 M Elsabbagh, G Divan, Y Koh, Y Shin Kim, S Kauchali, C Marcin, C Montiel-Nava, V Patel, C S Paula, C Wang, M Taghi Yasamy, E Fombonne. Global prevalence of autism and other pervasive developmental disorders. Autism Research (2012) 5: 160-179.

19 Centers for Disease Control and Prevention. Autism Spectrum Disorder (ASD). http://www.cdc.gov/ncbddd/autism/data.html

20 B S Abrahams, D H Geschwind. Advances in autism genetics: on the threshold of a new neurobiology. Nature Reviews Genetics (2008) 9(5): 341-355.

21 M K Belmonte, E H Cook Jr, G M Anderson, JLR Rubenstein, W T Greenough, A Beckel-Mitchener, E Courchesne, L M Boulanger, S B Powell, P R Levitt, E K Perry, Y H Jiang, T M DeLorey, E Tierney. Autism as a disorder of neural information processing: directions for research and targets for therapy. Molecular Psychiatry (2004) 9: 646-663.

22 Salvatore A Curenti. Understanding and determining the etiology of autism. Cellular and Molecular Neurobiology (2010) 30(2): 161-171.

23 Z Warren, J Veenstra-VanderWeele, W Stone, J L Bruzek, A S Nahmias, J H Foss-Feig, R N Jerome, S Krishnaswami, N A Sathe, A M Glasser, T Surawicz, M L McPheeters. Therapies for children with Autism spectrum disorders. http://www.nimh.nih.gov/health/publications/a-parents-guide-to-autism-spectrum-disorder/parent-guide-to-autism.pdf

24 R K Sharma and Bhagwan Dash. Caraka Samhita (text with English translation and critical exposition based on Cakrapani Datta's Ayurveda Dipika) volume 2. Chowkhamba Sanskrit Series Office, Varanasi, India, Reprint 2007.

25 Y Deepmala, B Banshidhar, K Abhimanyu. Probable etiopathogenesis (samprapti) of autism in frame of ayurveda in relation to intense world theory. Global J Res. Med. Plants & Indigen. Med. (2013) 2(6): 448-459.

26 K R Srikantha Murthy. Vagbhata's Astanga Hrdayam, Vol I (text, English translation, notes, appendices and indices). Chowkhamba Krishnadas Academy, Varanasi, India. Seventh edition, 2010. [p. 167]

27 S K Ramachandran, G Harini Ramya. Childhood autism intervention with certain Ayurvedic drugs and procedure based therapies. Government Ayurveda College, Thiruvanathapuram, India.

28 Mukesh Jain. Ayurvedic Treatment for Autism. http://health.sulekha.com/ayurvedic-treatment-for-autism_558568_blog

29 Prasad M. Ayurveda for Autism Spectrum Disorder. http://www.articlesbase.com/mental-health-articles/ayurveda-for-autism-spectrum-disorder-3343086.html

30 T Sandhya, J Sowjanya, B Veeresh. Bacopa monniera (L.) wettst ameliorates behavioral alterations and oxidative markers in sodium valproate induced autism in rats. Neurochemical Research (2012) 37(5): 1121-1131.

10 – Anticonvulsant Activity

10.1 – General

Epilepsy is a common, chronic brain disorder characterized by recurrent unprovoked seizures that are caused by abnormal electrical activity in the brain. Seizures are short episodes of uncontrolled behavior that can last anywhere from a few seconds to several minutes. They vary widely, from momentary lapses of attention and muscle jerks to severe and prolonged convulsions[1]. Most seizures fall under two broad categories: partial (or focal) seizures and generalized seizures[2]. Partial seizures begin in a localized region of the brain, whereas generalized seizures apparently start all over the brain. More than half of all observed epileptic disorders have no identifiable cause. The rest have been attributed to various factors including genetics, head trauma, stroke, heart disease, prenatal injury and developmental disorders[1]. Epilepsy affects nearly 50 million people worldwide, and more than 80 percent are in developing regions[1]. The mortality rate in epileptic patients is two to three times higher than in the general population[3]. There is no cure for epilepsy at present, but treatments are available to eliminate or reduce seizures. Conventional therapies utilize antiepileptic drugs (AEDs) and, occasionally, surgical therapy. AEDs satisfactorily control seizures in 60-70% of patients[1], but they can also cause adverse side effects.

10.2 – Ayurveda and Epilepsy

In Ayurveda, epilepsy is referred to as Apasmara or Apasmrti, and it is well-described in the literature[4]. The Charaka Samhita states that epilepsy is "characterized by frequent or occasional loss of consciousness associated with terrifying activities (vomiting of froth and abnormal movements of limbs) due to disturbance of the mind, intellect and other psychic faculties."[5] Epilepsy is classified into four major types based on the dominant dosha involved in the development of the disease: vataja (vata imbalance), pittaja (pitta imbalance), kaphaja (kapha imbalance) and sannipataja (imbalanced vata, pitta and kapha). Each type exhibits its own symptoms. Endogenous, exogenous and psychological factors are implicated in the cause of epilepsy[4]. A variety of strategies and formulations for the treatment of epilepsy are available in Ayurveda[6,7]. The anticonvulsant properties of a number of plants have been reported[8-11].

10.3 – Experimental Evidence

Rao and Karanth[12] investigated the effect of aqueous and alcoholic extracts of Bacopa monniera (whole plant) on maximal electroshock (MES) and pentylenetetrazole (PTZ) induced seizures in rats. Both an acute and a long term study (15 days) were conducted.

In the acute study with MES, neither the aqueous extract (0.3 or 0.6 g/kg, i.p.) nor the alcoholic extract (4 or 7 g/kg, i.p.) abolished any of the phases of MES. However, at the higher dose, both extracts decreased the duration of the extensor phase without much change in the flexor phase, indicating a reduction of seizure severity. In the long-term study, neither the aqueous extract (3 g/kg/day, PO) nor the alcoholic extract (2 g/kg/day, PO) showed any effect.

In the acute study with PTZ, rats treated with the aqueous extract (0.6 g/kg, i.p.) or the alcoholic extract (7 g/kg, i.p.) showed a delay in the onset of convulsions and no mortality. In the long-term study, both the aqueous extract (3 g/kg/day, PO) and the alcoholic extract (2 g/kg/day, PO) delayed the onset of convulsions with no mortality.

The investigators concluded that treatment with either extract may be beneficial in treating petit mal seizures, where a person loses awareness of their surroundings for up to 20 sec.

Shukia and coworkers[13] examined the anticonvulsant activity of Brahmi rasayana in rodents using the MES and PTZ models. Brahmi rasayana is a polyherbal formulation that contains Bacopa monniera. In the MES model (150 mA for 0.2 s), rats treated with Brahmi rasayana (3, 10 or 30 g/kg, PO) showed a decrease in the duration of the extensor phase compared to the control group. In the PTZ model (100 mg, SC), mice treated with Brahmi rasayana (3, 10 or 30 g/kg) showed a delay in the onset of convulsions, decreased duration of tonic seizures and reduced mortality compared to the control group.

Shanmugasundaram and coworkers[14] investigated the efficacy of Brahmigritham (BG), an Ayurvedic herbal formula, in controlling PTZ-induced seizures in rats. BG was made from Bacopa monniera and other herbs. Diazepam was also examined for comparison. Rats were treated with BG (0.5 mL/day, PO) or diazepam (2 mg/kg/day, PO) for a period of one week to four months and challenged with PTZ (250 mg/kg i.p.) after the last dose. The results are summarized below:

- Pretreatment of rats with BG or diazepam for three or more months prevented PTZ-induced seizures in all rats, while shorter periods of pretreatment were less effective or not effective at all.
- BG was as effective as diazepam in protecting rats against PTZ-induced seizures.
- BG did not depress neurological functions and electrical responses in the brain.

Achliya and coworkers[15] investigated the anticonvulsant activity of Unmadnashak ghrita (UG), using MES and PTZ models. UG, an Ayurvedic formulation, is composed of Bacopa monniera and other herbs. The results are summarized below:

- In the MES model, rats were treated with UG (100-500 mg/kg, PO) or saline (control) and subjected to MES (42 mA for 0.2 sec). The UG group showed a decreased tonic extensor phase compared to the control group. The effect was dose-dependent.
- In the PTZ model, rats were treated with UG (100-500 mg/kg, PO) or saline (control) and challenged with PTZ (70 mg/kg, SC). The UG group showed a delayed onset of the tonic phase and the tonic hindlimb extensor phase compared to the control group.

Balamurugan and coworkers[16] evaluated the antiepileptic activity of a polyherbal extract (PHE) containing Bacopa monniera. Adult Wistar albino rats (2-3 months old) treated with PHE (250 or 500 mg/kg/day, PO) or phenytoin (20 mg/kg/day, PO) for 15 days and subjected to MES (150 mA, 60 Hz, 0.2 s) showed the following changes compared to rats treated with the vehicle and subjected to MES:

- Reduction of various seizure phases and recovery time
- Increased levels of serotonin, dopamine and noradrenaline (forebrain)

The effect of PHE was comparable to phenytoin. The authors concluded that "**administration of PHE for 15 days increased the seizure threshold in MES-induced rats and its possible mechanism may be due to inhibition of prostaglandin synthesis and monoamine oxidase enzyme. One more possible mechanism involved in the antiepileptic effect of PHE may be by the decreased influx of calcium ions.**"

Kaushik and coworkers[17] demonstrated the anticonvulsant activity of an alcoholic extract of Bacopa monniera (BM) in rodents using different convulsive models: PTZ, MES, strychnine, hypoxic-stress and lithium-pilocarpine.

Khan and coworkers[18] evaluated the effect of an aqueous extract of Bacopa monniera (whole plant) on glutamate receptor binding and NMDAR1 gene expression in the hippocampus of epileptic rats. Glutamate is the primary excitatory neurotransmitter in the brain and acts through the NMDA receptors. Epilepsy was induced in adult male Wistar rats by administering pilocarpine (350 mg/kg, i.p.). The epileptic rats were divided into two groups. One group was treated with BM (300 mg/kg, PO) for 15 days. The other group was used as an epileptic control. A separate group of normal rats treated with the vehicle served as the normal control. Rats from each group (normal control, epileptic control and BM) were subjected to the Morris water maze test. The rats were sacrificed for hippocampal assay. The results are summarized below:

- In the Morris water maze test, the epileptic control group showed impairment of spatial memory compared to the normal control group. The BM group showed less impairment of spatial memory compared to the epileptic control group (close to the normal control group).
- The epileptic control group showed increased glutamate dehydrogenase activity, decreased glutamate binding, and decreased NMDAR1 gene expression compared to the normal control group. Treatment of epileptic rats with BM reversed these changes (close to the normal control group).

The investigators concluded that the "**BM extract potentiates a therapeutic effect by reversing the alterations in glutamate receptor binding and NMDAR1 gene expression that occur during epilepsy.**"

Paulose and coworkers[19] examined the effect of Bacopa monniera on metabotropic glutamate receptor 8 (mGluR8) gene expression in the cerebellum of epileptic rats. Activation of mGlu receptors is known to inhibit glutamate release. The experimental procedure was similar to the investigation described previously[18]. Rats from each group were assessed with the Morris water maze test daily. After the treatment period, the rats were sacrificed and the cerebellum was removed for analysis. The results are summarized below:

- In the Morris water maze task, the epileptic control group showed impairment of spatial memory compared to the normal control group. The BM group showed less impairment of spatial memory compared to the epileptic control group (close to the normal control group).
- The epileptic control group showed decreased mGluR8 gene expression in the cerebellum compared to the normal control

group. Treatment of epileptic rats with BM restored mGluR8 gene expression (close to the normal control group).

Krishnakumar and coworkers[20] investigated the effect of an aqueous extract of Bacopa monniera (BM) on 5-HT_{2c} receptors, 5-HT_{2c} gene expression, and inositol triphosphate (IP3) in the brain of epileptic rats, as well as on the behavioral changes associated with epilepsy. 5-HT_{2c} has been implicated in the cause of depression and other psychiatric disorders. IP3 has many functions, including the regulation of Ca^{2+}. The experimental procedure was similar to a previous study[18], with some modifications. The effect of carbamazepine (CBZ, 150 mg/kg/day, PO, 15 days) on epileptic rats was also examined. Rats from each group were subjected to the forced swim test daily. After the treatment period, the rats were sacrificed for biochemical analysis. The results are summarized below (Table 10.1):

Test/Assay	Epileptic control (2) compared to Normal control (1)	Epileptic + BM (3), Epileptic + CBZ (4) compared to Epileptic control (2)
Forced swim	Showed depressive behavior	Showed less depressive behavior
5-HT_{2c}, 5-HT_{2c} gene expression (hippocampus)	Upregulated	Downregulated
IP3 (cerebral cortex, hippocampus, cerebellum, brainstem)	Increased	Decreased

Table 10.1: Effects of BM on 5-HT_{2c} receptors in the hippocampus of pilocarpine-induced epileptic rats

The investigators stated that "**pilocarpine-induced temporal lobe epileptic rats have enhanced 5-HT_{2c} gene expression and receptor binding and increased IP3 content in hippocampus and associated depressive mood behavioral changes. BM treatment antagonized these effects, suggesting a therapeutic role in the management of epilepsy.**"

Mathew and coworkers[21] investigated the effect of Bacopa monniera and its active component bacoside A on GABA and $GABA_A$ receptors in the hippocampus of epileptic rats, as well as on the behavioral changes associated with epilepsy. GABA is the chief inhibitory neurotransmitter in the central nervous system. The experimental procedure was similar to the study described above[18], with some modifications. The effect of bacoside A (BA, 150 mg/kg/day, PO, 15 days) was also examined. Rats from each group were subjected to the radial maze and y-maze tests. The rats were then sacrificed for biochemical analysis. Major findings are summarized below (Table 10.2):

Test/Assay	Epileptic control (2) compared to Normal control (1)	Epileptic + BM (3), Epileptic + BA (4), Epileptic + CBZ (5) compared to Epileptic control (2)
Y-maze and radial maze	Showed decreased exploratory behavior and impairment in spatial memory and learning.	Showed improved exploratory behavior, spatial memory and learning.
Scatchard analysis (hippocampus)	GABA and $GABA_A$ receptors decreased	GABA and $GABA_A$ receptors increased
Glutamate decarboxylase (GAD) mRNA in the hippocampus	GAD mRNA downregulated	GAD mRNA upregulated (close to normal)

Table 10.2: Effects of BM, bacoside A and CBZ on behavior changes and GABA receptor functional regulation in the hippocampus of epileptic rats

The authors concluded that "**decreased GABA receptors and GAD activity in the hippocampus encompass an important role during seizure initiation and memory deficit associated with TLE (temporal lobe epilepsy) and Bacopa monnieri and its active component Bacoside-A is beneficial against memory impairment in epileptic rats.**"

Mathew and coworkers[22] investigated the effect of Bacopa monniera (BM) and bacoside A (BA) on metabolism and excitability in epileptic rats. The experimental procedure was similar to the previous study[21]. Group 2 showed increased serum T3 and insulin, muscle AChE and malate dehydrogenase (MDH), and decreased heart AChE compared to group 1. Groups 3, 4 and 5 showed a reversal of these changes. The authors suggested that "**repetitive seizures resulted in increased metabolism and excitability in epileptic rats. Bacopa monnieri and Bacoside-A treatment**

prevents the occurrence of seizures thereby reducing the impairment on peripheral nervous system."

Mathew and coworkers[23] investigated the effect of Bacopa monniera (BM) and bacoside A (BA) on GABAergic receptor binding and gene expression in the cerebral cortex, as well as on spatial learning and memory in epileptic rats. The experimental procedure was similar to a previous study[21]. Major findings are summarized below (Table 10.3):

Test/Assay	Epileptic control (2) compared to Normal control (1)	Epileptic + BM (3), Epileptic + B A (4), Epileptic + CBZ (5) compared to Epileptic control (2)
Y-maze and radial maze	Showed decreased exploratory behavior and impairment in spatial memory and learning	Showed improved exploratory behavior, spatial memory and learning.
Scatchard analysis (cerebral cortex)	GABA and $GABA_A$ receptors decreased	GABA and $GABA_A$ receptors increased
$GABA_B$, GAD65 and CREB mRNA (cerebral cortex)	$GABA_B$ and GAD65 mRNA showed downregulation; CREB mRNA showed upregulation	$GABA_B$ and GAD65 mRNA showed upregulation; CREB mRNA showed downregulation

Table 10.3: Effects of BM, bacoside A and CBZ on spatial learning and memory, GABAergic receptor binding and gene expression in the cerebral cortex of epileptic rats

The authors concluded that the study "**showed the therapeutic significance of Bacopa monnieri, and its active component Bacoside-A in the management of epilepsy, associated mood disorders and memory problems.**"

References

1 World Health Organization. Epilepsy, fact sheet No. 999. October 2012
2 Centers for Disease Control and Prevention. Epilepsy: Frequently Asked Questions. http://www.cdc.gov/epilepsy/basics/faqs.htm
3 A Gaitatzis, J W Sander. The mortality of epilepsy revisited. Epileptic Discord (2004) 6(1): 3-13.
4 S Jain, P N Tandon. Ayurvedic medicine and Indian literature on epilepsy. Neurology Asia (2004) 9 (supplement 1): 57-58.
5 R K Sharma and Bhagwan Dash. Caraka Samhita (text with English translation and critical exposition based on Cakrapani Datta's Ayurveda Dipika) volume 2. Chowkhamba Sanskrit Series Office, Varanasi, India, Reprint 2007.
6 Heena A Bhatt, Nithya J Gogtay, Sudeshna S Dalvi, Nilima A Kshirsagar. "Epilepsy" in Scientific Basis for Ayurvedic Therapies. Edited by Lakshmi Chandra Mishra. CRC Press, Boca Raton, FL, 2004.
7 Kumar Dileep, Kumar Sarvesh, Murthy K H H, V S S Narasimha. Ayurvedic formulations for the management of epileptic disorders. International Research Journal of Pharmacy (2012) 3(6): 17-20.
8 Lucindo J Quintans Jr, Jackson R G S Almeida, Julianeli T Lima, Xirley P Nunes, Jullyana S Siqueira, Leandra Eugenia, Gomes de Oliveira, Reinaldo N Almeida, Petronio F de Athayde-Filho, Jose M Barbosa-Filho. Plants with anticonvulsant properties - a review. Brazilian Journal of Pharmacognosy (2008) 18 (Supl.): 798-819.
9 Malvi Reetesh K, Bigoniya Papiya, Sethi Sunny, Jain Sonam. Medicinal plants used in the treatment of epilepsy. International Research Journal of Pharmacy (2011) 2(2): 32-39.
10 Suresh Kumar, Reecha Madaan, Gundeep Bansal, Anupam Jamwal, Anupam Sharma. Plants and plant products with potential anticonvulsant activity - a review. Pharmacognosy Communications (2012) 2(1, Supp 1): 3-99.
11 A G Nikalje, A Altamash, M S Ghodke. Herbal anticonvulsant agents: a brief review. International Journal of Research in Pharmacy and Science (2012) 2(3): 1-13.
12 Gladys Martis, A Rao, K S Karanth. Neuropharmacological activity of Herpestis monniera. Fitoterapia (1992) 63(5): 399-404.
13 Bina Shukia, N K Khanna, J L Godhwani. Effect of Brahmi rasayan on the central nervous system. Journal of Ethnopharmacology (1987) 21: 65-74.
14 E R B Shanmugasundaram, G K Mohammed Akbar, K Radha Shanmugasundaram. Brahmighritham, an Ayurvedic herbal formula for the control of epilepsy. Journal of Ethnopharmacology (1991) 33: 269-276.
15 Girish S Achliya, Sudhir G Wadodkar, Avinash K Dorle. Evaluation of sedative and anticonvulsant activities of unmadnashak Ghrita. Journal of Ethnopharmacology (2004) 94: 77-83.
16 G Balamurugan, P Muralidharan, S Selvarajan. Anti epileptic activity of poly herbal extract from Indian medicinal plants. Journal of Scientific Research

(2009) 1(1): 153-159.

17 Darpan Kaushik, Ashish Tripathi, Rashmi Tripathi, Madiwalayya Ganachari, Suroor Ahmad Khan. Anticonvulsant activity of Bacopa monniera in rodents. Brazilian Journal of Pharmaceutical Sciences (2009) 45(4): 643-649.

18 Reas Khan, Amee Krishnakumar, C S Paulose. Decreased glutamate receptor binding and NMDA R1 gene expression in hippocampus of pilocarpine-induced epileptic rats: neuroprotective role of Bacopa monnieri extract. Epilepsy & Behavior (2008) 12: 54-60.

19 C S Paulose, Finla Chathu, S Reas Khan, Amee Krishnakumar. Neuroprotective role of Bacopa monnieri extract in epilepsy and effect of glucose supplementation during hypoxia: glutamate receptor gene expression. Neurochem Res (2008) 33: 1663-1671.

20 Amee Krishnakumar, M S Nandhu, C S Paulose. Upregulation of 5-HT_{2C} receptors in hippocampus of pilocarpine-induced epileptic rats: antagonism by Bacopa monnieri. Epilepsy and Behavior (2009) 16: 225-230.

21 Jobin Mathew, Gireesh Gangadharan, Korah Kuruvilla, C S Paulose. Behavioral deficit and decreased GABA receptor functional regulation in the hippocampus of epileptic rats: effect of Bacopa monnieri. Neurochem Res (2011) 36(1): 7-16.

22 Jobin Mathew, Jes Paul, M S Nandhu, C S Paulose. Increased excitability and metabolism in pilocarpine induced epileptic rats: effect of Bacopa monnieri. Fitoterapia (2010) 81: 546-551.

23 Jobin Mathew, Savitha Balakrishnan, Sherin Anthony, Pretty Mary Abraham, C S Paulose. Decreased GABA receptor in the cerebral cortex of epileptic rats: effect of Bacopa monnieri and bacoside-A. Journal of Biomedical Sciences (2012) 19(1): 25.

11 – Immunomodulatory Activity

11.1 – General

Immunity is the general capacity of the body to overcome a specific infection or disease[1]. The immune system has an exceptional ability to distinguish between self and other. There are two types of immune responses: innate and adaptive. Innate immunity is the immunity with which a person is born. It provides an immediate, non-specific defense against invading toxins and pathogens. Adaptive immunity, also referred to as specific immunity, provides defense against particular invaders. Adaptive immunity improves with repeated exposure to foreign agents such as viruses, bacteria and toxins. Molecules that are capable of binding to the products of immune responses are called antigens, and the antigens that also elicit immune responses are called immunogens[2]. The terms antigen and immunogen are often used interchangeably. The immune system consists of a complex network of cells, tissues, organs and molecules that work together.

11.2 – Cells of the Immune System[1,3]

In adults, the cells responsible for immunity originate from the bone marrow. The pluripotent stem cells in the bone marrow divide to form two lineages: lymphoid stem cells and myeloid stem cells. Lymphoid stem cells differentiate to form lymphocytes: B cells, T cells, and natural killer cells. The myeloid stem cells differentiate into neutrophils, eosinophils, basophils, mast cells, monocytes, macrophages and dendritic cells. The progeny of the lymphoid and myeloid cells named above are collectively known as white blood cells (leukocytes).

11.2.1 – Neutrophils[1,4,5]

Neutrophils, also called polymorphonuclear leukocytes, are the most abundant type of circulating white blood cells. They are generated in the bone marrow in large numbers. An adult human produces about 10-20 billion new neutrophils per day, but they are short lived. Neutrophils are likely to be the first type of immune cells to arrive at the site of an infection. Neutrophils are phagocytes. When a phagocyte finds a pathogen, it engulfs the pathogen and creates a vesicle enclosing the pathogen called a phagosome. Lysosomes present in the cell then fuse with the phagosome to form a phagolysosome, which breaks down the pathogen. This process is called phagocytosis.

11.2.2 – Macrophages[1,6]

Monocytes mature in tissues to become macrophages. They are active phagocytes. After killing a pathogen by phagocytosis, they process the digested pathogen and display a small portion of the pathogen protein on the membrane surface in association with major histocompatibility complex II (MHCII). Macrophages are known as antigen-presenting cells (APCs). Macrophages release various cytokines, giving them a regulatory role in the immune response. Monocytes and macrophages also remove dead and dying cells.

11.2.3 – Dendritic Cells[1,7,8]

Dendritic cells comprise only a small fraction (0.2%) of the white blood cells in the body. They are phagocytes. Dendritic cells are efficient in processing phagocytized pathogens. They present a small portion of the pathogen protein on the membrane surface in association with MHCII. Dendritic cells are best known for their role in initiating T cell immunity.

11.2.4 – Eosinophils[1,9]

Eosinophils constitute about 1-5% of white blood cells. They contain a large number of tiny sacs called granules that are loaded with toxic chemicals. Once stimulated, eosinophils release those chemicals to kill pathogens that are too big for phagocytes.

11.2.5 – Basophils[1,10]

Basophils comprise less than 1% of circulating white blood cells. They contain a large number of granules, and upon stimulation release histamine, prostaglandin, serotonin and leukotrienes.

11.2.6 – Mast Cells[2,11]

Mast cells have granules that contain pharmacologically active compounds. They mediate inflammatory responses such as hypersensitivity and allergic reactions. Mast cells have been shown to be crucial for optimal immune responses during infection.

11.2.7 - Natural Killer Cells[1,12]

Natural killer cells (Nk) are a small population of large non-phagocytic granular lymphocytes. Their major function is to destroy cells that are malignant and infected with microorganisms. Nk cells inject the pore-forming protein performin into the plasma membrane of the target cell and release cytotoxic enzymes called granzymes.

11.2.8 - T Cells[1,6]

T cells, also known as T lymphocytes, are produced in the bone marrow and move to the thymus, where they mature. They have specific receptors (TCRs) on their plasma membrane surface. TCRs recognize antigen fragments exposed on the surfaces of antigen presenting cells (macrophages, dendritic cells and B cells) in association with MHCI and MHCII molecules. T cells are divided into two categories: regulatory cells and cytotoxic cells. Helper cells (T_H) are the most important type of regulatory T cells. When a naive T_H cell recognizes a specific antigen-MHCII complex, it is activated and undergoes proliferation and differentiation. These cells secrete numerous cytokines that can activate B cells, T cells and many other immune and nonimmune cells. T_H cells can differentiate into at least three functional classes which have unique cytokine profiles. Cytotoxic cells (T_C) kill virus-infected cells, transplanted tissues and cancer cells. T_C cells recognize antigen fragments on infected cells in association with the MHCI complex. T_C cells kill by injecting perforin and granzymes, or by a mechanism that leads to apoptosis.

11.2.9 - B Cells[1,6]

B cells, also known as B lymphocytes, originate and mature in the bone marrow. Each B cell can bind to a specific antigen, for which it deploys a large number of receptors on its surface (BCRs). Upon activation, B cells differentiate into plasma cells and memory B cells. Plasma cells produce antibodies (immunoglobulins). The various classes of antibodies (IgG, IgM, IgA, IgO and IgE) are related to membrane bound BCRs. Memory cells mediate quicker responses to subsequent infection by the same antigen.

Activation of B cells requires two steps. The first step occurs when a B cell encounters its specific antigen. BCRs bind to the antigen and internalize the antigen by endocytosis. The antigen is digested and a small fragment of the antigen is presented on the surface of the cell in association with MHC II molecules. The second step typically involves T cells. TCRs on helper T cells bind to the antigen-MHC II complex on the B cell, resulting in T cell activation. The activated T cell secretes numerous cytokines that activate the B cell. The second step can also occur independent of T cells, when some types of antigens activate the B cell directly.

11.3 – Ayurveda and Immunity

In Ayurveda, immunity is referred to as Vyadhikshamatva[13]. It literally means resistance to disease. A synonym for vyadhikshamatva is Bala (strength). The Charaka Samhita[14] mentions three types of bala - sahaja, kalaja and yuktikrita:

Trividham Balamithi - sahajam, kalajam, yuktikritam cha

- Sahaja (innate) – constitutional strength present since birth
- Kalaja (temporal) - strength depends on the time of day, season and age of the person
- Yuktikrita (acquired) – immunity acquired by various means during the lifetime

Ojas is considered to be the most important factor in imparting immunity to a person. Rasayana therapy with special herbs is prescribed to enhance immunity[15-17].

11.4 – Experimental Evidence

Sarapanchotiwitthaya and coworkers[18] examined the immunomodulatory activities of an alcohol extract of Bacopa monniera (BM) and bacoside A (BA) in mice. Splenocyte (white blood cells situated in the spleen) proliferation and phagocytic activities were determined.

Splenocyte proliferation activity was determined by the MTT technique. A suspension of splenocytes isolated from female ICR mice was treated with BM or BA with or without a mitogen (5 μg/mL). The following mitogens (substances that activate cell division) were used: lipopolysaccharides (LPS), pokeweed mitogen (PWM), phytohaemagglutinin (PHA) and Con A. Major findings are summarized below:

- BM suppressed splenocyte proliferation (SP) in the absence of a mitogen, as well as in the presence of LPS, PWM and PHA. With Con A, BM suppressed SP at lower doses, and stimulated SP at higher doses.
- BA stimulated SP in the absence of a mitogen, as well as in the presence of PWM and PHA. BA suppressed SP in the presence of LPS. With Con A, BM suppressed SP at lower doses, and stimulated SP at higher doses.

Phagocytic activity was determined by NBT dye reduction and lysosomal enzyme activity assays. Peritoneal mouse macrophages were treated with BM or bacoside A. Cellular lysosomal activity was determined by treating the macrophage suspension with BM or bacoside A. The results are summarized below:

- Both BM and BA showed a slight decrease in NBT reduction compared to the control group, indicating inhibition of $O_2^{\bullet -}$.
- BM (10 mg/mL) produced a slight increase in lysosomal enzyme activity compared to the control group, indicating weak phagocytic activation. The effect of BA was comparable to the control group.

The authors concluded that "**B. monniera manifests various effects on the murine immune system depending on the immune cell types.**"

Hule and Juvekar[19] investigated the effect of a saponin-rich fraction of Bacopa monniera (SRF) on the release of immune mediators from murine peritoneal exudate cells (PECs), as well as on the proliferation of immune cells. PECs were isolated from Swiss albino mice and cultured. These cells were treated with different concentrations of SRF (6.5 - 832 µg/mL). A number of assays were performed on the incubated cells, and the stimulation index (SI) was calculated. The following observations were made for PECs treated with SRF:

- Stimulated nitrite release (SI=2.14 at SRF=208 µg/mL). Nitrite production is an indicator of NO release, which is an index of macrophage activation.
- Stimulated and suppressed NBT dye reduction. SI values were 1.34 (SRF=52 µg/mL) and 0.67 (SRF=832 µg/mL).
- Increased lysosomal enzyme activity (SI=1.89 at SRF=104 µg/mL).
- Increased myeloperoxidase (MPO) activity (SI=1.43 at SRF=832 µg/mL). MPO uses H_2O_2 to convert Cl^- to HOCl (bactericidal agent)

A sulforhodamine B (SRB) assay was performed on isolated murine PECs, splenocytes and bone marow cells. The SRB assay is useful in screening cell viability/cytotoxicity in vitro. The proliferative index values were 1.56, 1.44 and 1.34 for PECs, splenocytes and bone marrow cells, respectively.

The authors concluded that an SRF "**containing triterpene saponin glycosides [is] able to activate murine peritoneal exudate cells (consisting mainly of macrophages and neutrophils), resulting in the increased production of various immune mediators and was able to stimulate viability of immune cells.**"

Juvekar and coworkers[20] evaluated the immunomodulatory activity of a methanol extract of Bacopa monniera. In vitro evaluation was done by measuring the mediators (nitric oxide and superoxide) released from murine peritoneal macrophages. Treatment of the cells with the extract stimulated the release of nitric oxide at 416 μg/mL (SI=1.67) and 208 μg/mL (SI=2.64). The extract-treated cells showed NBT reduction at 52 μg/mL (SI=1.34).

Yamada and coworkers[21] evaluated the immunomodulatory effects of Bacopa monniera (BM). Four-week old male Sprague Dawley rats were treated with a regular diet (control group) or a diet containing Bacopa monniera for four weeks. The rats were then sacrificed and blood was withdrawn from the abdominal aorta. Serum Ig concentration was measured. Spleen lymphocytes from both groups were isolated and cultured. These cells were incubated with or without Con A (10 μg/mL) or LPS (10 μg/mL) for 48 hours at 37 °C. A number of assays were performed on the incubated cells. Major findings from this investigation are summarized below:

- Rats fed with BM showed higher concentrations of serum IgA and IgG compared to the control group. Serum IgE and IgM did not significantly differ between the groups.
- Splenic lymphocytes of rats fed with BM showed higher levels of IgA, IgG, IgM, IL-2, IFN-γ and IL-6 compared to the control group. This occurred both in the presence and absence of mitogens (LPS or Con A).
- Splenic lymphocytes of rats fed with BM showed decreased levels of TNF-α compared to the control group. This occurred both in the presence and absence of mitogens.
- In the absence of mitogens, splenic lymphocytes of rats fed with BM showed no significant change in the level of IL-4 compared to the control group. In the presence of Con A, IL-4 levels increased. LPS had no effect on IL-4.

References

1 Lansing M Prescott, John P Harley, Donald A Klein. Microbiology, Fifth Edition. McGraw Hill, New York, 2005.
2 Abul K Abbas, Andrew H Lichtman. Cellular and Molecular Immunology, Fifth Edition. Saunders, Philadelphia, 2003.
3 P S Noakes, L J Michaelis. "Innate and adaptive immunity" in Diet, Immunity and Inflammation. Edited by Philip C Calder and Parveen Yaqoob, Elsevier, 2013.
4 Niels Borregaard. Neutrophils, from marrow to microbes. Immunity (2010) 33: 657-670.
5 V Kumar, A Sharma. Neutrophils: Cinderella of innate immune system. International Immunopharmacology (2010) 10: 1325-1334.
6 Klaus D Elgert. Immunology: Understanding the Immune System. John Wiley & Sons, 2009.
7 Ralph M Steinman. Dendritic cells: versatile controllers of the immune system. Nature Medicine (2007) 13(10): 7-11.
8 Jacques Banchereau. "The long arm of the immune system" in Scientific American (2002) November: 52-59.
9 C A Behm, K S Ovington. The role of eosinophils in parasitic helminth infections: insights from genetically modified mice. Parasitology Today (2000) 16(5): 202-209.
10 Brandon M Sullivan, Richard M Locksley. Basophils: a nonreductant contributor to host immunity. Immunity (2009) 30(1): 12-20.
11 Soman N Abraham, Ashley L St John. Mast cell-orchestrated immunity to pathogens. Nature Reviews Immunology (2010) 10(6): 440-452.
12 Xavier Camous, Alejandra Pera, Rafael Solana, Anis Larbi. NK cells in healthy aging and age-associated diseases. Journal of Biomedicine and Biotechnology (2012). doi: 10.1155/2012/195956
13 P S Byadgi. Concept of immunity in Ayurveda. Journal of Applied Pharmaceutical Science (2011) 1(5): 21-24.
14 R K Sharma and Bhagwan Dash. Caraka Samhita (text with English translation and critical exposition based on Cakrapani Datta's Ayurveda Dipika) volume 1. Chowkhamba Sanskrit Series Office, Varanasi, India, Reprint 2007.
15 Ashish A Mungantiwar, Aashish S Phadke. "Immunomodulation: therapeutic strategy through Ayurveda" in Scientific Basis for Ayurveda Therapies. Edited by Lakshmi Chandra Mishra. CRC press, Boca Raton, FL 2004.
16 K Gulati, A Ray, P K Debnath, S K Bhattacharya. Immunomodulatory Indian medicinal plants. Journal of Natural Remedies (2002) 2(2): 121-131.
17 K Singh, B Verma. The concept of vyadhikshamatva (immunity) in Ayurveda. International Journal of Ayurveda and Allied Sciences (2012) 1(5): 99-108.
18 Aurasorn Saraphanchotiwitthaya, Kornkanok Ingkaninan, Pattana Sripalakit. Effect of Bacopa monniera Linn. extract on murine immune response in vitro. Phytotherapy Research (2008) 22: 1330-1335.
19 A K Hule, A R Juvekar. In vitro immune response of saponin rich fraction of

Bacopa monnieri, Linn. International Journal of PharmTech Research (2009) 1(4): 1032-1038.

20 A Juvekar, M Juvekar, A Hule, S Wankhede. In vitro and in vivo immunomodulatory activity evaluation of Bacopa monniera, Scrophulariaceae. Planta Medica (2009) 75.

21 Koji Yamada, Pham Hung, Tae Kyu Park, Pyo Jam Park, Beong Ou Lim. A comparison of the immunostimulatory effects of the medicinal herbs Echinacea, Ashwagandha and Brahmi. Journal of Ethnopharmacology (2011) 137: 231-235.

12 – Anti-inflammatory Activity

12.1 – General

Inflammation is the body's normal response to harmful stimuli such as pathogens, toxic chemicals, injury or irritation. The inflammatory response involves dilation of blood vessels, increased blood flow, increased vascular permeability, exudation of fluids, and mediator release, among other responses[1]. It helps in neutralizing harmful stimuli and initiating the healing process[2]. However, if inflammation persists for a long time and is not treated, it may lead to disease[3]. The four cardinal signs of inflammation are redness, heat, swelling and pain.

12.2 – Ayurveda and Inflammation Disorders

Ayurveda recognizes inflammation as: "(a) symptom of a disease (b) independent disease and (c) a complication of diseases."[4]. Clinical features of Amavata, Sandhigata Vata and Rakta Vata in Ayurveda resemble the inflammatory disorders rheumatoid arthritis, osteoarthritis and gouty arthritis, respectively[5]. In Ayurveda, several plants, both alone and in combination, have been used to treat inflammation[3,5-10].

12.3 – Experimental Evidence

Jain and coworkers[11] investigated the anti-inflammatory activity of Brahmi rasayana (BR) against experimentally induced inflammation in rodents. BR is a polyherbal formulation whose major component is Bacopa monniera. Acute and sub-acute studies were conducted.

In the acute study, rats were treated with BR (1-10 g/kg, PO) or indomethacin (1-10 mg/kg, PO), and 30 minutes later were injected with carrageenan (0.1 mL of 1% solution) into the plantar aponeurosis of the right hind paw. Paw volume was measured before and 30 minutes after carrageenan administration. Similar experiments were also conducted with nystatin (0.1 mL of 6% solution). Paw volume was measured before and after nystatin administration at various intervals. Indomethacin, a nonsteroidal anti-inflammatory drug, was used as a standard reference. Both the BR and indomethacin groups showed comparable dose-dependent decreased paw edema. However, indomethacin was toxic at a higher dose (10 mg/kg).

Sub-acute inflammation was induced in rats by implanting two sponge pellets in the subcutaneous tissues on the back of the rat, one on each side of the midline. The rats were treated with BR (1-10 g/kg, PO) or indomethacin (1-10 mg/kg, PO) for six days and sacrificed on the 7th day. The pellets, along with granuloma tissues, were removed, dried and weighed. Both the BR and indomethacin groups showed less granular formation compared to the control group, but indomethacin was toxic at 10 mg/kg.

Experiments were also done using reserpinized rats in the carrageenan-induced inflammation studies. The results indicated that the anti-inflammatory activity of BR was not due to adrenergic factors.

The authors suggested that BR "**may partially mediate its antiinflammatory activity by interfering with the action and/or synthesis of prostaglandins and also perhaps by stabilization of the lysosomal membranes. Its anti-inflammatory activity is comparable to that of indomethacin.**"

Channa and coworkers[12] studied the effect of an alcoholic extract of Bacopa monniera (BM) against carrageenan-induced inflammation in mice and rats. Mice were treated with the vehicle, BM (100 mg/kg, i.p.) or aspirin (100 mg/kg, i.p.). After 30 minutes, carrageenan (30 µL, 1% vol/vol) was administered. The paws were amputated 3 hours later and weighed. Both BM-treated and aspirin-treated mice showed similar decreased paw edema compared to the control group.

Similar experiments were done with rats using different doses of BM (10-100 mg/kg, i.p.) or aspirin (10-100 mg/kg, i.p.) and 50 µL of carrageenan. At 10 mg/kg, neither the BM group nor the aspirin group showed any detectable effect on paw edema compared to the control group. However, at 50 or 100 mg/kg, both groups showed reduced paw edema. BM was more effective than aspirin.

Experiments were also done to discern the anti-inflammatory mechanism of BM. The results showed that BM did not inhibit inflammation induced by histamine, serotonin or bradykinin, whereas chlorpheniramine inhibited histamine and methysergide inhibited serotonin-induced inflammation. BM inhibited prostaglandin-induced inflammation. Caffeic acid inhibited arachidonic acid-induced inflammation, whereas BM and aspirin had no effect.

The authors concluded that "**the ethanol extract of Bacopa monniera possesses strong anti-inflammatory activity via prostaglandin inhibition**".

Viji and Helen[13] evaluated the anti-inflammatory activity of different Bacopa monniera preparations against carrageenan-induced inflammation in rats. An ethanol extract of Bacopa monniera (BME) was most effective among the preparations at inhibiting edema in rats induced by carrageenan. Monocytes from rats treated with BME or voveran and injected with carrageenan showed decreases in 5-LOX and 15-LOX activities compared to monocytes from untreated rats injected with carrageenan. BME was more effective than voveran. BME also inhibited COX-2 activity and was more effective than indomethacin.

In vitro studies using rat blood monocytes showed that the EtOAc fraction was most effective at inhibiting 5-LOX and 15-LOX activities. The EtOAc and bacoside-enriched fractions inhibited COX-1 and COX-2 activities. The ratio of the IC_{50} values for COX-1 to COX-2 inhibition was 9.09 and 11.81 for the EtOAc and bacoside-enriched fractions, respectively, indicating selective inhibition of COX-2. The corresponding value for indomethacin was 1.35. Both fractions also inhibited the release of the pro-inflammatory cytokine TNF-α in intravenous human blood activated by LPS.

The authors concluded that "**Bacopa monniera possesses anti-inflammatory activity through inhibition of COX and LOX and downregulation of TNF-α.**"

Viji and coworkers[14] investigated the effect of a methanol extract of Bacopa monniera (BM) on arthritis as well as on several inflammatory mediators and immune functions in rats. Arthritis was induced in male Wistar rats by the intradermal injection of bovine type II collagen dissolved in acetic acid and emulsified with incomplete Freund's adjuvant. This was followed by a booster shot after 7 days. Arthritic rats were treated with BM (100 mg/kg/day, PO) or indomethacin (3 mg/kg/day, PO) for 46 days starting from the 14th day after arthritic induction. Untreated normal rats and arthritic rats served as the normal control and arthritic control, respectively. The results are summarized below (Table 12.1):

Measurement	Arthritic control compared to Normal control	Arthritic + BM, Arthritic + Indomethacin, compared to Arthritic control
Paw size	Increased	Decreased; BM was more effective than indomethacin.
5-LOX activity in blood mononuclear cells	Higher	Lower
COX activity (paw tissue)	Higher	Lower; BM showed 87% COX-2 and 13% COX-1 inhibition. Indomethacin showed 11% COX-2 and 89% COX-1 inhibition.
MPO activity (articular cartilage)	Higher	Lower
Serum IgM and IgG	Higher	Lower; BM was more effective than indomethacin.
Histopathological study (knee joint) of the arthritic control group showed disrupted architecture, whereas arthritic rats treated with BM showed less disrupted architecture.		

Table 12.1: Effects of BM on arthritis, some inflammatory mediators and immune functions

The authors concluded that BM "**possesses remarkable antiarthritic activity.**"

Viji and Helen[15] examined the effects of triterpenoid and bacoside-enriched fractions prepared from a methanol extract of Bacopa monniera on pro-inflammatory mediator release in vitro, as well as on carrageenan-induced paw edema and adjuvant-induced arthritis in vivo.

In the in vitro study, human peripheral blood mononuclear cells (hPBMCs) were incubated with varying concentrations (0-25 μg/mL) of the triterpenoid or bacoside-enriched fraction and stimulated with LPS. LPS stimulation of hPBMCs without the triterpenoid or bacoside-enriched fraction increased the levels of TNF-α, IL-6 and MDA, and decreased SOD activity. In the presence of the triterpenoid or bacoside-enriched fraction, levels of TNF-α, IL-6 and MDA decreased. The triterpenoid fraction showed no significant effect on SOD activity, whereas the bacoside-enriched fraction reduced SOD activity. Mouse peritoneal exudate cells (PECs) treated with the triterpenoid or bacoside-enriched fraction inhibited nitrite production.

In the in vivo study, male Wistar rats were treated with the vehicle (control), triterpenoid fraction, or bacoside-enriched fraction, and carrageenan was injected. Rats treated with the triterpenoid or bacoside-enriched fraction showed decreased paw edema compared to the control group. The triterpenoid fraction was more effective.

The anti-arthritic acitivty of the triterpenoid fraction was also studied with an adjuvant model. Normal mice treated with the vehicle served as a normal control (group 1). Arthritis was induced by injecting Freund's complete adjuvant into the right hind paw of Swiss albino mice. The mice were then divided into two groups. One group (group 2) was used as an arthritic control, and the other group (group 3) was treated with the triterpenoid fraction (25 mg/kg, PO). The triterpenoid fraction was administered for 30 days starting on the day after the induction of arthritis. Foot pad thickness was measured during the experimental period. At the end of the experimental period, the mice were sacrificed and serum was isolated for analysis. Group 3 showed decreased paw edema (day 30), serum C-reactive protein (CRP), serum glutamate oxaloacetate transaminase (GOT) activity, and glutamate pyruvate transaminase (GPT) activity compared to group 2. Group 3 showed similar results to group 1.

The authors concluded that the study "**provides an insight into the ability of Bacopa monniera to inhibit inflammation through modulation of pro-inflammatory mediator release.**"

Viji and coworkers[16] examined the effect of Bacopa monniera on lysosomal instability in arthritic rats. A methanol extract of Bacopa monniera (BM) and a chloroform fraction (CF) prepared from the extract were used. Arthritis was induced in male Wistar rats by injecting complete Freund's adjuvant into the right hind paw. Arthritic (AIA) rats were treated with BM (100 mg/kg, PO), CF (50 mg/kg, PO), or indomethacin (3 mg/kg, PO). Untreated normal rats and AIA rats served as the normal control and AIA control, respectively. The results are summarized below:

- The AIA control group showed increased lysosomal enzyme activity and glycosaminoglycan in articular cartilage, and decreased hexose, hexuronic acid and sialic acid in synovial effusate compared to the normal control group. AIA rats treated with BM or indomethacin showed a reversal of these changes.
- The AIA control group showed increased Prostaglandin E_2 (PGE_2) in paw tissue and IL-6 expression in blood mononuclear

cells compared to the normal control group. AIA rats treated with CF or indomethacin showed a reversal of these changes.

- Paw tissues of the AIA control group showed severe inflammation, whereas AIA rats treated with CF showed less inflammation.

The authors concluded that "**the possible mechanism of action of the B. monniera extract may be through its stabilizing action on lysosomal membranes and hence the decrease in spread of inflammation.**"

Helen and coworkers[17] investigated (in vitro) the effect of betulinic acid on LPS-induced IL-6 production in hPBMCs. Betulinic acid (BA) was isolated from Bacopa monniera. LPS activation of cells increased IL-6 production. Cells pretreated with BA, a p38 inhibitor, or an ERK 1/2 inhibitor showed relatively decreased IL-6 after LPS activation. A JNK inhibitor showed no effect. Pretreatment of cells with BA along with both p38 and ERK 1/2 inhibitors was more effective at inhibiting IL-6 production than any one of them alone. LPS activation of cells caused nuclear translocation of p65 NF-κB, a feature that was not observed in unactivated cells. The nuclear extract of cells treated with BA, p38 or ERK 1/2 inhibitors showed decreased p65 after LPS activation compared to untreated cells. The nuclear extract of cells treated with BA, along with both p38 and ERK 1/2 inhibitors showed a further decrease in p65. Overall, the decrease in IL-6 production after LPS activation in cells treated with BA correlated with the inhibition of p65 NF-κB nuclear translocation.

In vivo studies showed that rats treated with BA for 7 days survived longer after LPS administration compared to untreated rats. Also, blood mononuclear cells of rats treated with BA showed downregulation of IL-6 after LPS administration compared to mononuclear cells from untreated rats.

The investigators concluded that "**the possible mechanism by which betulinic acid exerts anti-inflammatory effect included inhibition of IL-6 production via inhibition of NF-κB or p38/ERK MAPK pathway.**"

In a subsequent investigation, Helen and coworkers[18] examined the effect of BA on pro-inflammatory mediators produced by LPS activation of hPBMCs (in vitro). Pretreatment of hPBMCs with BA inhibited the production of PGE_2 and COX-2 gene expression. Cells pretreated with an ERK inhibitor or a P13K inhibitor decreased LPS-induced PGE_2 production, whereas a p38 inhibitor and a JNK inhibitor showed no significant effect. LPS stimulation of cells induced phosphorylation of Akt, ERK 1/2 and p38 MAPK. Pretreatment with BA inhibited LPS-induced phosphorylation of Akt and ERK 1/2, without affecting p38 MAPK phosphorylation. Cells pretreated with BA, an ERK inhibitor, or a P13K inhibitor inhibited LPS-induced nuclear translocation of NF-κB. BA also inhibited LPS-induced LDH release and ROS production in hPBMCs.

An in vivo study showed that pretreatment of mice with BA (20 mg/kg/day, i.p.) for 3 days before the administration of LPS (32 mg/kg, i.p.) enhanced the lifespan of mice and decreased PGE_2 and MPO in liver and lung tissues. BA pretreatment also prevented lung and liver injury induced by LPS.

The authors concluded that **"BA inhibits the inflammatory responses in LPS-stimulated hPBMCs. The anti-inflammatory effects of BA may be mediated by decreased COX-2 protein production and PGE_2 formation via the modulation of Akt and ERK and the subsequent down-regulation of NF-κB signalling. In addition, BA markedly reduced LPS-induced PGE_2 production in mouse liver and lungs."**

Padmanabhan and Jangle[1] demonstrated (in vitro) the anti-inflammatory activity of HP-4, a polyherbal preparation containing Bacopa monniera. HP-4 (100-500 μg/mL) inhibited protein denaturation and protected erythrocyte membranes against lysis induced by a hypotonic solution. The effect of HP-4 (500 μg/mL) was similar to acetylsalicylic acid (200 μg/mL).

Volluri and coworkers[19] showed that a methanol extract of Bacopa monniera (BM, 50–2000 μg/mL) inhibited protein denaturation and protected human red blood cell membranes. The effect of BM (2000 μg/mL) was similar to diclofenac sodium (2000 μg/mL).

References

1 P Padmanabhan, S N Jangle: Evaluation of in-vitro anti-inflammatory activity of herbal preparation, a combination of four medicinal plants. International Journal of Basic and Applied Medical Sciences (2012) 2(1): 109-116.

2 Juan Jesus Carrero, Peter Stenvinkel. Persistent inflammation as a catalyst for other risk factors in chronic kidney disease: a hypothesis proposal. Clinical Journal of the American Society of Nephrology (2009) 4: S49-S55.

3 Sekhar Shailasree, Karmakar Ruma, K Ramachandra Kini, Siddapura Ramachandrappa Niranjana, Harischandra Sripathy Prakash. Potential anti-inflammatory bioactives from medicinal plants of Western Ghats, India. Pharmacognosy Communications (2012) 2(2): 2-12.

4 P N Vinaya. Inflammation in Ayurveda and modern medicine. International Ayurvedic Medical Journal (2013) 1(4): 1-7.

5 Lakshmi Chandra Mishra. "Rheumatoid arthritis, osteoarthritis and gout" in Scientific Basis for Ayurveda Therapies. Edited by Lakshmi Chandra Mishra. CRC press, Boca Raton, FL, 2004.

6 M S Premila. Ayurvedic Herbs: a clinical guide to the healing plants of

traditional Indian medicine. The Haworth press Inc, Binghamton, NY, 2006.

7 K L Soeken, S A Miller, E Ernst. Herbal medicines for the treatment of rheumatoid arthritis: a systematic review. Rheumatology (2003) 42: 652-659.

8 Kushagra Nagori, Mukesh Kumar Singh, Dhansay Dewangan, V K Verma, D K Tripathi. Anti-inflammatory activity and chemo profile of plants used in traditional medicine: a review. Journal of Chemical and Pharmaceutical Research (2010) 2(5): 122-130.

9 S Agnihotri, S Wakode, A Agnihotri. An overview of anti-inflammatory properties and chemo-profiles of plants used in traditional medicine. Indian Journal of Natural Products and Resources (2010) 1(2): 150-167.

10 Talha Jawaid, Deepa Shukla, Jaiendra Verma. Anti-inflammatory activity of the plants used in traditional medicines. International Journal of Biomedical Research (2011) 2(4): 252-263.

11 P Jain, N K Khanna, N Trehan, V K Pendse, J L Godhwani. Antiinflammatory effects of an Ayurvedic preparation, Brahmi rasayan in rodents. Indian Journal of Experimental Biology (1994) 32: 633-636.

12 Shabana Channa, Ahsana Dar, Shazia Anjum, Muhammad Yaqoob, Atta-ur-Rahman. Anti-inflammatory activity of Bacopa monniera in rodents. Journal of Ethnopharmacology (2006) 104: 286-289.

13 V Viji, A Helen. Inhibition of lipoxygenases and cyclooxygenase-2 enzymes by extracts isolated from Bacopa monniera (L.) wettst. Journal of Ethnopharmacology (2008) 118: 305-311.

14 V Viji, S K Kavitha, A Helen. Bacopa monniera (L.) wettst inhibits type II collagen-induced arthritis in rats. Phytother. Res. (2010) 24: 1377-1383.

15 V Viji, A Helen. Inhibition of pro-inflammatory mediators: role of Bacopa monniera (L.) wettst. Inflammopharmacology (2011) 19(5): 283-281.

16 Viji Vijayan, G L Shyni, A Helen. Efficacy of Bacopa monniera (L.) wettst in alleviating lysosomal instability in adjvant-induced arthritis in rats. Inflammation (2011) 34(6): 630-638.

17 V Viji, B Shobha, S K Kavitha, M Ratheesh, K Kripa, A Helen. Betulinic acid isolated from Bacopa monniera (L.) wettst suppresses lipopolysaccharide stimulated interleukin-6 production through modulation of nuclear factor-κB in peripheral blood mononuclear cells. International Immunopharmacology (2010) 10: 843-849.

18 Vijayan Viji, Antony Helen, Varma R Luxmi. Betulinic acid inhibits endotoxin-stimulated phosphorylation cascade and pro-inflammatory prostaglandin E_2 production in human peripheral blood mononuclear cells. British Journal of Pharmacology (2011) 162: 1291-1303.

19 Sharan Suresh Volluri, Srinivasa Rao Bammidi, Seema Chaitanya Chippada, Meena Vangalapati. In-vitro anti-arthritic activity of methanolic extract of Bacopa monniera. International Journal of Chemical, Environment and Pharmaceutical Research (2011) 2(2-3): 156-159.

13 – Antistress Activity

13.1 – General

Stress is a part of normal life that most people experience at one time or another. The word 'stress' is often used to describe feelings towards situations that range from trivial to catastrophic. The same situations may elicit substantially different reactions in different people[1]. What one feels as a minor inconvenience may be felt as major stress by another, which makes stress a difficult concept to define. Hans Selye[2], a pioneer in stress research, defined stress as "the nonspecific response of the body to any demand". Recently, Koolhaas and coworkers[3] have proposed that "the term stress should be restricted to conditions where an environmental demand exceeds the natural regulatory capacity of an organism, in particular situations that include unpredictability and uncontrollability".

When a situation is perceived as a threat, it triggers a series of responses from several physiological systems. The sympathetic-adrenal-medullary (SAM) system and the hypothalamic-pituitary-adrenal (HPA) axis are considered to be the two most important pathways that mediate the stress response[4]. Activation of these pathways results in the release of glucocorticoids (corticosterone or cortisol) and catecholamines (adrenaline and noradrenaline) into the bloodstream[5]. These hormones enable the body to effectively respond and adapt to demanding internal and external stimuli. Glucocorticoids and catecholamines regulate a variety of physiological processes. Prolonged and repeated activation of the SAM and HPA systems can increase the risk for physical and psychiatric disorders[6].

13.2 – Ayurveda and Stress

In Ayurveda, stress is referred to as "Sahasa", and is recognized as contributing to the development of a number of diseases[7]. Stress depletes ojas and makes the body vulnerable. Ayurveda employs a number of stress management strategies that include proper lifestyle and the use of rasayanas. A number of herbs that have antistress potential have been reported.[8,9]

13.3 – Experimental Evidence

Chowdhuri and coworkers[10] examined the antistress activity of bacosides of Bacopa monniera (BBM) in rats. Stress was induced by cold-hypoxic restraint. Male Sprague Dawley rats treated with distilled water for 7 days and subjected to stress on day 7 (stress control) showed the following changes compared to rats treated with distilled water and not subjected to stress (normal control):

- Increased heat shock polypeptide 70 (Hsp 70) expression, 7-ethoxyresourfin-O-deethylase (EROD) and 7-pentoxyresorufin-O-dealkylase (PROD) activities in all brain regions studied
- Decreased SOD activity in the hippocampus without significant change in the other areas

Rats treated with BBM (20 or 40 mg/kg/day, PO) for 7 days and subjected to stress on day 7 showed decreased Hsp 70 expression and PROD activity in all brain regions studied compared to the stress control group. SOD and EROD activities increased, decreased or were unchanged depending on the brain region and concentration of BBM. The authors concluded that **"BBM has potential to modulate the activities of Hsp70, P450 [dependent enzymes EROD and PROD] and SOD thereby possibly allowing the brain to be prepared to act under adverse conditions such as stress."**

Rai and coworkers[11] investigated the antistress effect of a Bacopa monniera extract (BM) in rats using acute stress (AS) and chronic stress (CS). The effect of Panax quinquefolium (PQ) was also examined for comparison. Stress was applied by restraining individual rats in an acrylic hemicylindrical tube for 150 min. In the AS study, Sprague Dawley rats were treated with the vehicle (group 2), BM (40 or 80 mg/kg/day, PO; group 3), or PQ (100 mg/kg/day, PO; group 4) for 3 days and subjected to stress on the 3rd day. A group of rats treated with the vehicle and not subjected to stress served as a control (group 1). In the CS study, rats were treated in a similar manner for 7 days and stress was applied daily. Major findings are summarized below:

<u>AS Experiments</u>

- Group 2 showed increases in ulcer index, adrenal gland weight, plasma glucose, ALT, AST and CK, as well as decreased spleen weight compared to group 1.
- Group 3 (BM=40 mg) showed decreases in ulcer index, adrenal gland weight, plasma glucose, AST and CK compared to group 2. Group 3 (BM=80 mg) showed decreased adrenal gland weight,

plasma glucose, ALT, AST and CK, and increased spleen weight compared to group 2.

- Group 4 showed decreased plasma ALT, AST and CK, and increased spleen weight compared to group 2.

CS Experiments

- Group 2 showed increases in ulcer index, adrenal gland weight, plasma AST and CK, and decreased spleen weight, thymus weight, plasma triglycerides and cholesterol compared to group 1.
- Group 3 (BM=40 mg) showed decreases in ulcer index and plasma AST, and increased plasma glucose compared to group 2. Group 3 (BM=80 mg) showed decreases in ulcer index, adrenal gland weight, plasma AST and CK compared to group 2.
- Group 4 showed decreases in ulcer index, adrenal gland weight, plasma AST and CK compared to group 2.

The authors concluded that BM attenuates the HPA axis and is an effective antistress agent in both AS and CS, whereas PQ attenuates the HPA axis and is effective only in CS.

Sheikh and coworkers[12] examined the effect of a Bacopa monniera extract (BM) on stress-induced alterations in plasma corticosterone and brain noradrenaline (NA), dopamine and serotonin in rats. The effect of PQ was also examined for comparison. The experimental design was similar to the one described previously[11,] with some modifications. Instead of CS, chronic unpredictable stress (CUS) was applied. The stressors included immobilization, forced swimming, overnight soiled cage bedding, foot shock, day-night reversal and fasting. Major findings from this study are summarized below:

AS Experiments

- Group 2 showed increased plasma corticosterone, DA (cortex), 5-HT (cortex and hippocampus), and decreased NA (cortex and hippocampus) and DA (hippocampus) compared to group 1.
- Group 3 showed a reversal of the changes in group 2, except that there was no change in NA (cortex and hippocampus).
- Group 4 showed a reversal of the changes in group 2, except that there was no change in DA (hippocampus).

CUS Experiments

- Group 2 showed decreased NA (cortex and hippocampus), DA (cortex and hippocampus) and 5-HT (cortex and hippocampus), and increased plasma corticosterone compared to group 1.
- Group 3 showed a reversal of the changes in group 2, except that there was no change in DA (hippocampus).
- Group 4 showed a reversal of the changes in group 2, except that there was no change in DA (hippocampus).

The authors concluded that "**the adaptogenic activity of BM might be due to the normalization of stress induced alteration in plasma corticosterone and levels of monoamines like NA, 5-HT and DA in cortex and hippocampus regions of the brain, which are more vulnerable to stressful conditions analogous to the effects of PQ.**"

Anju[13] studied the antistress activity of an ethanol extract of Bacopa monniera (BM) in mice. Panax ginseng (PG) was also studied for comparison. Adult male Swiss albino mice (8 weeks old) treated with PG (100 mg/kg/day, PO) or BM (27 mg/kg/day, PO) for 7 days and subjected to the swim endurance test on day 8 showed longer swim durations compared to mice treated with distilled water, indicating the antistress activity of PG and BM. Mice treated with distilled water for 7 days and subjected to cold restraint stress on day 8 showed increased adrenal gland weight, plasma cortisol, total white blood cell (WBC) count, blood glucose, and serum triglycerides compared to the control group. Mice treated with PG or BM for 7 days and subjected to stress on day 7 showed a reversal of these changes. The authors concluded that "**the ethanolic extract of Bacopa monnieri possesses a potent adaptogenic activity.**"

Bharathi and coworkers[14] examined the antistress effect of Vedic Calm, a polyherbal formulation whose major component is Bacopa monniera. Withania somnifera (Ashwagandha), a well-known antistress herb, was also studied for comparison. Albino Wistar rats subjected to cold-immobilization stress showed increased WBC, serum glucose, AST, ALT, cholesterol, ulcer index, adrenal gland weight and liver weight, and decreased spleen weight compared to the control group. Rats pretreated with Vedic Calm (135 mg/kg/day, PO) or Withania somnifera (100 mg/kg/day, PO) for 10 days and subjected to stress showed a reversal in these changes.

References

1 L I Pearlin. "The social contexts of stress: in Handbook of Stress: Theoretical and Clinical Inspects. Edited by Leo Goldberger, Shimo Breznitz. The Free press, New York, 1982.

2 H Selye. Forty years of stress research: prinicpal remaining problems and misconceptions. CMA Journal (1976) 115: 53-56.

3 J M Koolhaas, A Bartolomucci, B Buwalda, S F de Boer, G Flugge, S M Korte, P Meerlo, R Murison, B Olivier, P Palanza, G Richter-Levin, A Sgoifo, T Steimer, O Stiedl, G Van Dijk, M Wohr, E Fuchs. Stress revisited: A critical evaluation of the stress concept. Neuroscience and Biobehavioral Reviews (2011) 35: 1291-1301.

4 S H Scharf, M V Schmidt. Animal models of stress vulnerability and resilience in translational research. Curr Psychiatry Rep (2012) 14(2): 159-165.

5 W Beerling, J M Koolhaas, A Ahnaou, J A Bouwknecht, S F de Boer, P Meerlo, W H I M Drinkenburg. Physiological and hormonal responses to novelty exposure in rats are mainly related to ongoing behavioral activity. Physiology and Behavior (2011) 103: 412-420.

6 Sheldon Cohen, Denise Janicki-Deverts, Gregory E Miller. Psychological stress and disease. JAMA (2007) 298(14): 1685-1687.

7 Deepa Arora, Mukesh Kumar, S D Dubey, S K Baapat. Stress-management: leads from Ayurveda. Ancient Science of Life (2003) 23(1): 8-15.

8 Pawar Vinod S, Hugar Shivakumar. A current status of adaptogens: natural remedy to stress. Asian Pacific Journal of Tropical Disease (2012) 2: S480-S490.

9 P Venkatesh, K M Rao, M Gobinath, G Umadevi, R Anitha, K A Kumar, K Sudharsan. A review on anti-stress activity of medicinal drugs from herbal sources. J. Pharm. Res. Dev. (2012) 1(1): 1-11.

10 D Kar Chowdhuri, D Parmar, P Kakkar, R Shukla, P K Seth, R C Srimal. Antistress effects of bacosides of Bacopa monnieri: modulation of Hsp70 expression, superoxide dismutase and cytochrome P450 activity in rat brain. Phytotherapy Research (2002) 16: 639-645.

11 Deepak Rai, Gitika Bhatia, Gautam Palit, Raghwendra Pal, Satyawan Singh, Hemant K Singh. Adaptogenic effect of Bacopa monniera (Brahmi). Pharmacology, Biochemistry and Behavior (2003) 75: 823-830.

12 Naila Sheikh, Ausaf Ahmad, Kiran Babu Siripurapu, Vijaya Kumar Kuchibhotla, Satyawan Singh, Gautam Palit. Effect of Bacopa monniera on stress induced changes in plasma corticosterone and brain monoamines in rats. Journal of Ethnopharmacology (2007) 111: 671-676.

13 Anju. Bacopa monnieri – a preliminary study evaluating its anti-stress activity in Swiss albino mice. Research Journal of Pharmaceutical, Biological and Chemical Sciences (2011) 2(4): 786-794.

14 K N Bharathi, N Sivaramaiah, Chowdary G Nagarjuna, A V S S S Gupta. Evaluation of antistress, anxiolytic and hypnotic activity of Vedic Calm, a polyherbal formulation. Pharmacognosy Magazine (2009) 5(19): 124-130.

14 – Antidiabetic Activity

14.1 – General

Diabetes is a chronic disorder of carbohydrate, fat and protein metabolism. Diabetes can be caused by reduced insulin production, resistance to insulin, or both. Insulin is a hormone produced by the pancreas that enables cells to absorb glucose from the bloodstream and produce energy. When insulin is deficient or ineffective, glucose accumulates in the blood, which can lead to heart disease, stroke, nerve damage and other serious health problems. In 2011, the number of diabetic people reached 366 million globally and is estimated to reach 552 million by 2030[1]. It is projected that diabetes will be the 7th leading cause of death in 2030[2].

There are three major types of diabetes. In type 1 diabetes, the pancreas produces little or no insulin. It can occur at any stage, but is most often diagnosed in children, teens or young adults. Treatment includes proper diet, exercise and daily insulin injections. Type 2 diabetes results from the body's ineffective use of insulin. It occurs most often in adults, but teens are increasingly being diagnosed with it. Type 2 diabetes comprises about 90% of the people with diabetes worldwide. Treatment includes proper diet, exercise and in a large number of cases, oral hypoglycemic agents and/or insulin. The third type is gestational diabetes, which is high blood sugar that develops during pregnancy. Symptoms are similar to type 2 diabetes.

14.2 – Ayurveda and Diabetes

In Ayurveda, diabetes is considered to be a Maharoga (major disease) in the category of Prameha, a complex group of disorders characterized by profuse urination. The Charaka Samhita, Sushruta Samhita and Ashtanga Hridaya describe the causes, symptoms, complications and treatment of prameha[3-5]. There are 20 subtypes of prameha, which are classified by the dominant dosha that is imbalanced: kapha (10 subtypes), pitta (6 subtypes) and vata (4 subtypes). Features of kapha and vata prameha resemble those of diabetes mellitus. If these types of prameha are not managed properly, they lead to Madhumeha ("sugary urine"), a serious condition[6,7]. In Ayurveda, type 1 diabetes is described as Sahaja (hereditary) and type 2 diabetes is described as Apathya Nimittaja (acquired)[8]. Ayurveda emphasizes diet (Ahar), lifestyle (Vihar) and medicine (Aushadha) in the management of diabetes. Plant-based medicines have been the mainstay of Ayurvedic diabetic treatments. Recently, a number of papers on antidiabetic plants with clinical/experimental data have appeared[8-13].

14.3 – Experimental Evidence

Ghosh and coworkers[14] demonstrated the antidiabetic effect of an ethanol extract of Bacopa monniera (BM) in diabetic rats. Glibenclamide (GC), an antidiabetic drug, was also studied for comparison. Diabetes was induced in Wistar albino rats by administering alloxan (150 mg/kg, i.p.) in normal saline. Both single dose and multiple dose studies were conducted. In the single dose study, normal and diabetic rats were treated with water, BM (300 mg/kg, PO) or GC (600 mg/kg, PO). Blood glucose levels of normal rats treated with BM were similar to untreated normal rats, indicating the absence of hypoglycemic activity. Diabetic rats treated with BM or GC showed lower blood glucose levels compared to untreated diabetic rats.

In the multidose study, diabetic rats were treated with water, BM (300 mg/kg/day, PO) or GC (600 mg/kg/day, PO) for 10 days. The body weights of the diabetic control group were lower than their day 1 values, whereas the weights of diabetic rats treated with BM or GC were higher than their day 1 values. Treatment of diabetic rats with BM or GC lowered blood glucose levels. Diabetic rats showed increased LPO and decreased GSH, CAT and SOD in the liver compared to the control group. Treatment with BM or GC reversed these changes.

In vitro studies showed that BM inhibited hemoglobin glycosylation and increased peripheral glucose consumption similar to insulin. The authors concluded that the antihyperglycemic effect of BM might be due to increased peripheral glucose consumption as well as protection against oxidative damage in alloxanized diabetes.

In a subsequent investigation, Ghosh and coworkers[15] showed the antihyperglycemic activity of bacosine in alloxan-induced diabetic rats. Bacosine, a triterpene, was isolated from an ethanol extract of Bacopa monniera. Experiments similar to those described previously were done[14]. The results are summarized below:

- Normal rats treated with bacosine did not show significant changes in blood glucose levels compared to the normal control group, indicating the absence of hypoglycemic activity.
- In both the single and multiple dose studies, diabetic rats treated with bacosine (25 mg/kg) showed lower blood glucose levels com-

pared to the corresponding diabetic control group. The effect was comparable to glibenclamide (600 mg/kg).

- The diabetic control group showed weight loss during the experimental period, whereas the diabetic rats treated with bacosine gained weight.
- Livers of the diabetic control group showed increased LPO and decreased GSH, CAT, SOD and glycogen compared to the normal control group. Treatment with bacosine reversed these changes.

In vitro studies of hemoglobin glycosylation in the presence of various concentrations of bacosine showed inhibition of glycosylation in a dose-dependent manner. The IC_{50} value of bacosine (7.44 mg/mL) was comparable to α-tocopherol (7.74 mg/mL). Also, bacosine increased peripheral glucose consumption in the diaphragm of diabetic rats.

References

1 Kaivan Khavandi, Halima Amer, Bashar Ibrahim, Jack Brownrigg. Strategies for preventing type 2 diabetes: an update for clinicians. Therapeutic Advances in Chronic Disease (2013) 4(5): 242-261.

2 World Health Organization. Diabetes: fact sheet no. 312. March 2013.

3 R K Sharma and Bhagwan Dash. Caraka Samhita (text with English translation and critical exposition based on Cakrapani Datta's Ayurveda Dipika) volume 2. Chowkhamba Sanskrit Series Office, Varanasi, India, Reprint 2007.

4 K R Srikantha Murthy. Illustrated Susruta Samhita Vol II. Chaukhambha Orientalia, Varanasi, India, reprint 2010.

5 K R Srikantha Murthy. Vagbhata's Astanga Hrdayam (text, English translation, notes, appendices and indices) volume 2. Chowkhamba Krishnadas Academy, Varanasi, India. Seventh edition, 2010.

6 Hari Sharma, H M Chandola. Ayurvedic concept of obesity, metabolic syndrome and diabetes mellitus. The Journal of Alternative and Complementary Medicine (2011) 17(6): 549-552.

7 Hari Sharma, H. M. Chandola. Prameha in Ayurveda: Correlation with Obesity, Metabolic Syndrome, and Diabetes Mellitus. Part 1-Etiology, Classification, and Pathogenesis. The Journal of Alternative and Complementary medicine (2011) 17(6): 491-496.

8 Lakshmi Chandra Mishra, Tarek Adra. "Diabetes mellitus (madhumeha)" in Scientific Basis for Ayurvedic Therapies. Edited by Lakshmi Chandra Mishra. CRC Press, Boca Raton, FL, 2004.

9 M S Premila. Ayurvedic Herbs: a clinical guide to the healing plants of traditional Indian medicine. The Haworth press Inc, Binghamton, NY, 2006.

10 Manisha Modak, Priyanjali Dixit, Jayant Londhe, Saroj Ghaskadbi, Thomas Paul A Devasagayam. Indian herbs and herbal drugs used for the treatment

of diabetes. J. Clin. Biochem. Nutr. (2007) 40: 163-173.

11 Sarita Singh, Sunil Kumar Gupta, Gulam Sabir, Manish Kumar Gupta, Prahlad Kishore Seth. A database for anti-diabetic plants with clinical/experimental trials. Bioinformation (2009) 4(6): 263-268.

12 Akash Jain, Rishu Sharma, Nidhi Gahalain, Jasmine Chaudary, Girish Kumar Gupta. Herbal plants used in diabetic complications. an overview. Journal of Pharmacy Research (2011) 4(4): 986-988.

13 Farog Tayyab, Sapna Smith Lal, Meenakshi Mishra, Umesh Kumar. A review: medicinal plants and its impact on diabetes. World Journal of Pharmaceutical Research (2012) 1(4): 1019-1046.

14 Tirtha Ghosh, Tapan Kumar Maity, Pinaki Sengupta, Deepak Kumar Dash, Anindya Bose. Antidiabetic and in vivo antioxidant activity of ethanolic extract of Bacopa monnieri Linn. aerial parts: a possible mechanism of action. Iranian Journal of Pharmaceutical Research (2008) 7(1): 61-68.

15 Tirtha Ghosh, Tapan Kumar Maity, Jagadish Singh. Antihyperglycemic activity of bacosine, a triterpene from Bacopa monnieri, in alloxan-induced diabetic rats. Planta Med (2011) 77: 804-808.

15 – Antiulcer Activity

15.1 – General

Peptic ulcer disease (PUD) is one of the most common disorders of the gastrointestinal tract. A peptic ulcer is an open sore on the lining of the stomach (gastric ulcer) or the beginning of the small intestine (duodenal ulcer)[1,2]. Each year, more than half a million new cases of PUD are observed and more than one million people are hospitalized[3]. An estimated 25 million Americans are affected by PUD at some point in their lifetime.

The two major causes of PUD are Helicobacter pylori (H. pylori) infection and the long-term use of nonsteroidal anti-inflammatory drugs (NSAIDs) such as aspirin and ibuprofen[4]. H. pylori is a spiral-shaped bacterium that lives in the lining of the stomach. It causes more than 90% of duodenal ulcers and up to 80% of gastric ulcers. More than half of the world's population is infected with H. pylori, but most of them do not develop ulcers[5]. With PUD, there is an imbalance between offensive (acid, pepsin, H. pylori) and defensive mucosal factors (bicarbonate, nitric oxide, and growth factors).

Therapy for H. pylori infection includes antibiotics to kill the bacteria, proton pump inhibitors or histamine blockers to reduce stomach acid, and a bismuth-containing agent to protect the stomach and duodenal lining. Treatment for NSAID-induced PUD typically involves proton pump inhibitors or histamine blockers[5]. These drugs have side effects that include allergic reactions to acid-labile food proteins and drug hypersensitivity reactions[6].

15.2 – Ayurveda and PUD

In Ayurveda, PUD is known as Parinamasula[7]. Parinama means digestion and sula means sharp pain. Parinamasula represents a disease characterized by piercing pain in the abdomen which is felt during the digestion of food. The Madhava Nidana[8] and Bhavaprakasha[9] have described this Vyadhi (disease). Parinamasula is a tridoshaja vyadhi – all three doshas (vata, pitta, and kapha) are involved[7]. According to the Bhavaprakasha, vata gets aggravated and hinders the action of pitta and kapha, giving rise to pain in the abdomen during digestion. Ayurveda offers effective treatment for parinamasula, which includes a variety of herbs. Several plants have been investigated for antiulcer activity[10-19].

15.3 – Ulcer Models

The antiulcer activity of Bacopa monniera has been demonstrated by a number of investigators in a variety of ulcer models. These models are briefly described below.

15.3.1 – Ethanol[20,21]

The administration of absolute alcohol to rodents induces reproducible gastric lesions. Rats are fasted for 24-36 hours followed by the administration of 95-99% alcohol at a dose of 1 mL/200 g body weight. After 1 hour, the animals are sacrificed and the stomach is isolated for ulcer examination.

15.3.2 – NSAID[20-22]

NSAIDs primarily induce gastic ulcers by suppressing prostaglandin synthesis. Rats are fasted for 24-36 hours followed by oral administration of an NSAID (such as aspirin). After 4 hours, the animals are sacrificed and the stomach is isolated for ulcer examination.

15.3.3 – Cold-restraint Stress (CRS)[20,21]

The combination of restraint with low temperature induces gastric ulcers in rodents. Rats are fasted for 18 hours and strapped on a wooden plank kept at 4-6 °C for 2 hours. The animals are then sacrificed and the stomach is isolated for ulcer examination.

15.3.4 – Pyloric ligation (PL)[20-22]

Ulceration is caused by the accumulation of acidic gastric juice in the stomach. The rats are fasted for 18 hours and anesthetized with pentobarbitone. The abdomen is opened and the pylorus is ligated. The abdomen is then sutured. The animals are deprived of water during the postoperative period. After 4 hours of pyloric ligation, the animals are sacrificed. The stomach is cut open for content collection and ulcer examination.

15.3.5 – Acetic Acid[20-22]

This model resembles human ulcers in many ways. It is used in screening potential antiulcer drugs. After the rats are anesthetized, the abdomen is opened and the stomach is exposed. A glass tube containing acetic acid (50%, 0.06 mL) is placed in contact with the gastric wall for 60 seconds. The acid is then removed and the abdomen is closed. 24 hours later, the animals are sacrificed and the stomach is cut open for ulcer examination.

15.3.6 – Cysteamine[20,23,24]

Cysteamine-induced duodenal ulcers have been widely used as a model of PUD. Cysteamine-induced ulcers resemble human duodenal ulcers in many ways. The mechanism of cysteamine-induced ulcerogenesis may involve increased gastrin and gastric acid production, decreased gastric emptying and inhibition of bicarbonate and mucus production. Duodenal ulcers are induced by administering cysteamine (40 mg/200 g, PO) twice, at intervals of four hours. Afterwards, rats are allowed to drink only water containing cysteamine (0.05%). After 24 hours, the animals are sacrificed. The stomach along with 5 cm of the duodenum are taken out. The stomach is cut along the lesser curvature down to the duodenum for ulcer examination.

15.3.7 – Hydrochloric Acid[24]

Hydrochloric acid induces ulcers by increasing stomach acidity. Rats are deprived of food but not water for 18 hours. Hydrochloric acid (0.6 N, 1 mL) is administered orally.

15.4 – Experimental Evidence

Rao and coworkers[25] examined the antiulcer activity of a fresh juice of Bacopa monniera (BMJ) in rats using various gastric ulcer models. Sucralfate (SFT), an antiulcer drug, was also examined for comparison. CF albino rats were divided into three main groups and treated for 5 days (twice daily) as follows:

Group	Treatment
1	Distilled water (control)
2	BMJ (100 or 300 mg/kg/day, PO)
3	SFT (250 mg/kg/day, PO)

Gastric ulcers were induced in all groups on day 6 with ethanol, aspirin, CRS or PL, and the animals were then sacrificed. BMJ (300 mg) or SFT (250 mg) showed a similar decrease in ulcer index in all models. Both BMJ and SFT groups showed decreased DNA content in gastric juice, indicating less gastric mucosal damage (cell shedding) compared to the control group. The BMJ and SFT groups showed increased mucin concentration (indicator of mucosal resistance) compared to the control group. The authors attributed the antiulcer activity of BMJ to its effects on mucosal defensive factors.

Sairam and coworkers[21] studied the prophylactic as well as curative effects of a methanol extract of Bacopa monniera (BME) against experimentally induced gastric ulcers in rats. To study the prophylactic effect, CF albino rats were treated with the vehicle (control), BME (10-50 mg/kg/day, PO) or SFT (250 mg/kg/day, PO) for 5 days. On day 6, ulcers were induced with ethanol, aspirin, CRS or PL. The BME and SFT groups showed a dose-dependent decrease in ulcer index compared to the control group. The effect of BME at 50 mg was comparable to SFT. The BME group (20 mg) showed decreased volume, concentration, and output of acid and pepsin compared to the control group. The BME group also showed less mucosal damage compared to the control group.

The curative effect of BME was investigated by inducing ulcers in rats with acetic acid and treating them with the vehicle (control) or BME (20 mg/kg/day, PO) for 5 or 10 days. The BME group showed a decrease in ulcer index compared to the control group after 5 days. After 10 days, significant decreases in ulcer index and perforations were observed. Rats treated with BME and subjected to CRS showed a decrease in ulcer index and LPO, and an increase in SOD and CAT compared to rats treated with the vehicle and subjected to CRS. The authors suggested that the antioxidant activity of BME may be one of the important factors responsible for the anti-ulcerogenic activity of BME.

Dorababu and coworkers[24] investigated the ulcer protective and healing activity of a methanol extract of Bacopa monniera (BME) in normal rats and rats with non-insulin dependent diabetes mellitus (NIDDM). NIDDM was induced by administering streptozotocin (STZ, 70 mg/kg, i.p.) to 5-day-old rat pups. The standard antiulcer drugs sucralfate (SFT) and ranitidine (RAN), along with the anti-diabetic drug glibenclamide (GLC), were also examined for comparison. In ulcer protective studies, normal and NIDDM rats were treated orally for 6 days with the vehicle (control), BME (50 mg/kg/day), SFT (500 mg/kg/day), RAN (2.5 mg/kg/day) or GLC (0.6 mg/kg/day). On day 6, animals were subjected to ulceration. Gastric ulcers were induced ethanol, aspirin, CRS or PL. Duodenal ulcers were induced with cysteamine. NIDDM rats showed a greater tendency for ulceration compared to normal rats in all models of gastric and duodenal ulceration. BME showed ulcer protective activity in both NIDDM and normal rats, but was more effective in normal rats. Both SFT and RAN exhibited ulcer protective activity. GLC did not show significant ulcer protective activity in normal rats, but showed a moderate effect in diabetic rats.

For ulcer healing studies, normal and NIDDM rats were subjected to ulceration with acetic acid or HCl. They were treated as before. The HCl group was treated for 5 days and the acetic acid group for 10 days. The results are summarized below:

- BME treatment healed ulcers induced by acetic acid and HCl in both normal and NIDDM rats.
- Treatment with SFT and RAN also healed ulcers induced by acetic acid and HCl. SFT and RAN were more effective in the normal group than in the NIDDM group.
- Treatment with GLC healed acetic acid-induced ulcers in the NIDDM group only, but showed healing capacity in HCl-induced ulcers in both the NIDDM and normal groups.

Bafna and Balaraman[26] studied the anti-ulcer activities of DHC-1 in rats. DHC-1 is a polyherbal formulation that contains Bacopa monniera. PL and ethanol were used to induce ulcers. Female Wistar albino rats were treated with the vehicle or DHC-1 (125-1000 mg/kg, PO) and subjected to PL. After 19 hours, the rats were sacrificed. Rats treated with the vehicle and not subjected to ulceration served as a control group. In the ethanol-induced ulcer model, rats were treated with the vehicle or DHC-1 (125-1000 mg/kg/day, PO) for 10 days and subjected to ulceration with ethanol one hour later. The animals were then sacrificed. The results for both models are summarized below:

- Rats treated with DHC-1 and subjected to ulceration showed a dose-dependent decrease in ulcer index, volume of gastric fluid and total acidity compared to rats treated with the vehicle and subjected to ulceration.
- Rats treated with the vehicle and subjected to ulceration showed increased LPO and decreased SOD, CAT, GSH, Na^+/K^+-ATPase, Ca^{2+}-ATPase and Mg^{2+}-ATPase compared to the control group. Rats treated with DHC-1 showed a reversal in these changes.

The authors concluded that **"DHC-1 possesses anti-ulcer activity, which can be attributed to its antioxidant mechanism of action."**

Goel and coworkers[27] investigated the effect of a methanol extract of Bacopa monniera (BME) on H. pylori activity and the accumulation of prostaglandins. The NCTC 12822 strain of H. pylori was used. The effect of bismuth subcitrate (BSC), an inhibitor of H. pylori, was also examined.

H. pylori (NCTC 12822) was incubated with or without BME (1000 mg/mL) or BSC (1000 mg/mL) in a growth medium under a microaerophilic atmosphere. Both BME and BSC inhibited 75% of the growth of H. pylori compared to the control group.

An in vitro study of the effect of BME on the accumulation of prostanoids was done using human colonic tissues. Human colonic mucosal pieces were incubated with or without BME (0.1-10 μg/mL) or indomethacin (0.1-10 μg/mL). Indomethacin reduced the concentrations of both PGE and PGI_2 compared to the control group, whereas BM (10 μg/mL) increased the concentration of both PGE (40.8%) and PGI_2 (50.5%).

References

1 H. Pylori and Peptic ulcers. NIH Publication No 10-4225, National Digestive Diseases Information Clearinghouse (NDDIC), Bethesda, MD, 2010.

2 Theodore W Schafer. Peptic ulcer disease. http://patients.gi.org/topics/peptic-ulcer-disease/

3 Helicobacter pylori and peptic ulcer disease. http://cdc.gov/ulcer/keytocure.htm

4 NSAIDs and peptic ulcers. National Digestive Diseases Information Clearinghouse, Bethesda, MD (2010). NIH Publication No.10-4664

5 Peter Malfertheiner, Francis K L Chan, Kenneth E L McCall. Peptic ulcer disease. The Lancet (2009) 374(9699): 1449-1461.

6 E Ramirez, R Cabanas, L S Laserna, A Fiandor, H Tong, N Prior, O Calderon, N Medrano, I Bobolea, J Frias, S Quirce. Proton pump inhibitors are associated with hypersensitivity reactions to drugs in hospitalized patients: a nested case-control in a retrospective cohort study. Clinical & Experimental Allergy (2013) 43(3): 344-352.

7 S P Gandhi, R H Singh. A critical study of the concept of amlapitta and parinamasula. Ancient Science of Life (1993) 23(1-2): 111-118.

8 Umesananda Sarma. Madhava Nidana of Sri Madhavakara with the Sudhalahari Comments. by Pt. Sri Umesananda Sara, Edited by Brahma Sankara Sastri. Chowkhamba Sanskrit Series Office. Benares, India, 1943.

9 K R Srikantha Murthy. Bhavaprakasha of Bhavamisra. Chowkhamba Krishnadas Academy, Varanasi, India. Fourth edition 2009.

10 Krishnamurthy Sairaman, Sailaja Vani Batchu. "Gastroduodenal ulcers" in Scientific Basis for Ayurvedic Therapies. Edited by Lakshmi Chandra Mishra. CRC Press, Boca Raton, FL, 2004.

11 M S Premila. Ayurvedic Herbs: a clinical guide to the healing plants of traditional Indian medicine. The Haworth Press Inc, Binghamton, NY, 2006.

12 M Umashankar, S Shruti. Traditional Indian herbal medicine used as antipyretic, antiulcer, anti-diabetic and anticancer: a review. International Journal of Research in Pharmacy and Chemistry (2011) 1(4): 1152-1159.

13 S Sen, R Chakraborty, B De, J Mazumder. Plants and phytochemicals for peptide ulcer: an overview. Pharmacognosy Review (2009) 3(6): 270-279.

14 H S Falcao, I R Mariath, M F F M Diniz, L M Batista, J M Barbosa-Filho.

Plants of the American continent with antiulcer activity. Phytomedicine (2008) 15(1): 132-146.

15 M Rupesh Kumar, Mohamed Niyas K, T Tamizh Mani, O M Fasalu Rahiman, Satya Kumar B. A review on medicinal plants for peptic ulcer. Der Pharmacia Lettre (2011) 3(2): 180-186.

16 Ananya Chatterjee, Sirshendu Chatterjee, Sandip K Bandyopadhyay. H. pylori-induced gastric ulcer: pathophysiology and herbal remedy. IJBMR (2012) 3(1): 1461-1465.

17 Agrawal Krishn Kumar, Singh Kishan, Verma Anju, Singh Kuldeep. A review of ulcer healing plants. Novel Science-IJPS (2012) 1(8): 515-528.

18 J M Joy, AVS P Kumar, S Mohanalakshmi, C K Ashok Kumar, G A K Reddy, S Prathyusha. A review on anti-ulcer medicinal plants. International Journal of Pharmacology and Toxicology (2012) 2(2): 95-103.

19 R Patel, T Jawaid, P Gautam, P Dwivedi. Herbal remedies for gastroprotective action: a review. International Journal of Phytopharmacy (2012) 2(2): 30-38.

20 M B Adinortey, C Ansah, I Galyuon, A Nyarko. In vivo models used for evaluation of potential anti-gastroduodenal ulcer agents. Hindawi Publishing Corporation (2013). doi: 10.1155/2013/796405

21 K Sairam, Ch V Rao, M Dora Babu, R K Goel. Prophylactic and curative effects of Bacopa monniera in gastric ulcer models. Phytomed (2001) 8(6): 423-430.

22 Shawon Lahiri, Gautam Palit. An overview of the current methodologies used for evaluation of gastric and duodenal anti-ulcer agents. Pharmacologia (2012) 3(8): 249-257.

23 S Boesby, W K Man, R Mendez-Diaz, J Spencer. Effect of cysteamine on gastroduodenal mucosal histamine in rat. Gut (1983) 24(10): 935-939.

24 M Dorababu, T Prabha, S Priyambada, V K Agrawal, N C Aryya, R K Goel. Effect of Bacopa monniera and Azadirachta indica on gastric ulceration and healing in experimental NIDDM rats. Indian Journal of Experimental Biology (2004) 42(4): 389-397.

25 Ch V Rao, K Sairam, R K Goel. Experimental evaluation of Bacopa monniera on rat gastric ulceration and secretion. Indian Journal of Physiology and Pharmacology (2000) 44(4): 435-441.

26 P A Bafna, R Balaraman. Anti-ulcer and antioxidant activity of DHC-1, a herbal formulation. Journal of Ethnopharmacology (2004) 90(1): 123-127.

27 R K Goel, K Sairam, M Dora Babu, I A Tavares, A Raman. In vitro evaluation of Bacopa monniera on anti-helicobacter pylori activity and accumulation of prostaglandins. Phytomedicine (2003) 10(6): 523-527.

16 – Liver and Kidney Protective Activity

16.1 – General

The liver is the largest internal organ of the body, and has a number of vital functions that include[1]:

- Production of bile
- Metabolism of carbohydrate, protein and fat
- Conversion of glucose to glycogen
- Storage of glycogen, vitamins and minerals
- Synthesis of plasma proteins, blood coagulation factors and very low density proteins
- Detoxification and elimination of toxic substances

Exposure of the liver to toxic substances can lead to serious conditions like hepatitis, cirrhosis and hepatic cancer.

The kidneys are highly specialized organs that play an important role in regulating the volume and composition of extracellular fluid. They maintain a stable internal environment by selectively excreting appropriate amounts of various substances according to specific bodily needs. The kidneys have a variety of functions that include[1]:

- Fluid balance regulation
- Blood plasma ion concentration regulation
- Blood pressure and pH control
- Waste product elimination
- Hormone production

Many different conditions can affect kidney function. Most kidney problems are associated with other diseases such as diabetes or hypertension.

16.2 – Ayurveda and Liver and Kidney Disorders

In Ayurveda, the liver is called Yakrut. The Charaka Samhita, Sushruta Samhita and Ashtanga Hridaya have described kamala (jaundice) in the context of Pandu Roga (anemia)[2,3,4]. The Ashtanga Hridaya has also described kamala as a separate disease. In Ayurveda, the term Vrkka refers to the kidneys. The Sushruta Samhita and Ashtanga Hridaya have described various disorders of the kidneys and urinary tract. A number of plants are used in Ayurveda for the treatment of liver and kidney disorders[5-11].

16.3 – Liver and Kidney Toxicity Models

The effect of Bacopa monniera on liver and kidney toxicity in rats has been investigated by a number of researchers. A variety of chemical agents (listed below) have been used to induce liver and kidney toxicity.

16.3.1 – Acetaminophen (paracetamol)[12,13]

Acetaminophen is a popular antipyretic and analgesic found in over the counter and prescription drugs. It is generally safe at recommended doses, but overdose causes liver damage. In the liver, acetaminophen undergoes conjugation, and the conjugated metabolites are excreted in the urine. However, a small amount of acetaminophen produces toxic metabolites by a different metabolism. In the case of acetaminophen overdose, more toxic metabolites are produced, causing hepatic damage.

16.3.2 – D-Galactosamine (D-GAIN)[12,14]

D-GAIN is used extensively for inducing liver injury in experimental animals. It produces a diffuse type of liver injury that resembles human viral hepatitis. D-GAIN produces hepatotoxicity by depleting the uridine pool in hepatocytes.

16.3.3 – N-Nitrosodiethylamine (DEN)[15]

DEN, a well-known N-Nitrososalkyl compound, is a potent hepatotoxin and hepatocarcinogen. It can induce reproducible tumors after repeated administration. DEN is hydroxylated to α-hydroxylnitrosamine and after cleavage of acetaldehyde, an electrophilic ethyldiazonium ion is formed. This ion causes DNA damage. In addition, DEN causes oxidative stress.

16.3.4 – Nitrobenzene[16,17]

Nitrobenzene is a major industrial chemical. It is a hazardous air pollutant and a proven carcinogen in animals. Any means of exposure to nitrobenzene can result in toxicity to multiple organs. In mammals, three primary mechanisms of metabolism have been identified: reduction to aniline by intestinal microflora, reduction by hepatic microsomes in erythrocytes, and oxidative metabolism by hepatic microsomes. The metabolic processes are important because the toxic effects of nitrobenzene are triggered by its metabolites.

16.3.5 – Morphine[18,19]

Morphine is a potent analgesic and is extensively used in the management of severe acute and chronic pain. Morphine is metabolized essentially in the liver, gastrointestinal tract and kidneys. It is known to cause liver and kidney toxicity. The adverse reactions of morphine have been associated partly with the generation of reactive metabolites that can bind to GSH.

16.3.6 – Gentamicin[20,21]

Gentamicin, an aminoglycosidic antibiotic, is used in the treatment of severe infections. Although effective, its usefulness is limited because it can cause ototoxicity and nephrotoxicity. Gentamicin accumulates in renal proximal tubules, damaging brush border integrity. Other factors that contribute to pathogenesis include generation of free radicals in kidneys, diminishing of the antioxidant defense system, acute tubular necrosis, and glomerular congestion.

16.3.7 – Cisplatin[20,22]

Cisplatin is an anticancer drug. Its main dose-limiting side effect is nephrotoxicity associated with its accumulation in the kidneys. The mechanism of cisplatin-induced toxicity includes inflammation, oxidative stress, DNA damage, mitochondrial dysfunction, ATP depletion, glutathione depletion, and induction of apoptosis.

16.4 – Experimental Evidence

Sumathi and coworkers[23] investigated the hepatoprotective effect of an alcohol extract of Bacopa monniera (BMA) in rats against morphine-induced liver toxicity. Rats treated with morphine (50 mg/kg/day, i.p.) for 10 days showed increased LPO and decreased SOD, CAT, GPx, GRX and GSH in the liver compared to the control group. Rats treated with morphine and BMA (40 mg/kg/day, PO) for 10 days showed a reversal of these changes. The authors concluded that the "**Bacopa monniera alcohol extract exerted a hepatoprotective effect against morphine induced liver toxicity.**"

Ghosh and coworkers[24] examined the effect of an ethanol extract of Bacopa monniera (EBM) on acetaminophen-induced damage in rat liver cells. Rats treated with acetaminophen (500 mg/kg/day, PO) for 7 days showed the following changes compared to the control group:

- Decreased liver weight
- Increased serum GOT, GPT, alkaline phosphatase (ALP), bilirubin and total cholesterol
- Decreased liver GSH, SOD, CAT and LPO

Rats treated with acetaminophen and EBM (300 mg/kg/day, PO) or silymarin (25 mg/kg/day, PO) for 7 days showed a reversal of these changes. The authors suggested that the hepatoprotective effect of EBM might be due to its ability to restore the antioxidants depleted by acetaminophen.

Sumathi and Ramakrishnan[25] studied the hepatoprotective effect of an alcohol extract of Bacopa monniera (BME) against D-GAIN-induced liver injury in rats. Rats treated with the vehicle for 7 days and injected with a single dose of D-GAIN (400 mg/kg, i.p.) on the 7th day showed the following changes compared to the control group:

- Increased serum ALT, AST, LDH, ALP and γ-glutamyl transferase (γGT)
- Decreased glucose-6-phosphatase, GSH, SOD, CAT, GPx and GR

Rats treated with BME (40 mg/kg/day, PO) for 7 days and injected with a single dose of D-GAIN on the 7th day showed a reversal of these changes. The authors suggested that "**Bacopa monniera has hepatoprotective effect against D-GAIN induced hepatotoxicity.**"

Sumathi and Nongbri[26] investigated the hepatoprotective effect of bacoside A (BA) against D-GAIN-induced liver injury in rats. Rats treated with the vehicle for 21 days and injected with a single dose of D-GAIN (300 mg/kg, i.p.) on day 22 showed increased serum ALT, AST, LDH, ALP, γGT, LDH, 5'-nucleotidase, and decreased vitamin C and E in the plasma and liver compared to the control group. Rats treated with BA (10 mg/kg/day, PO) for 21 days and injected with D-GAIN on day 22 showed a reversal of these changes. The authors concluded that "**this study presents strong evidence of hepatoprotective effects of BA against D-GAIN intoxicated rats.**"

Janani and coworkers[27] examined the effects of bacoside A on DEN-induced liver toxicity in rats. Male adult albino rats treated with the vehicle for 14 days and injected with a single dose of DEN (200 mg/kg, i.p.) on day 15 showed the following changes compared to the control group:

- Decreased body weight and increased liver weight
- Increased liver LPO and ROS
- Decreased liver GSH, SOD, CAT, GPx, GR and GST
- Increased serum AST, ALT, LDH, ALP and γGT
- Loss of liver architecture

Rats treated with BA (15 mg/kg/day, PO) or silymarin (100 mg/kg/day, PO) for 14 days and injected with DEN on day 15 showed a reversal of these changes. The authors concluded that "**the present study highlights the protective effect of bacoside A on DEN-induced oxidative stress, which may be involved in the free radical scavenging mechanism.**"

Menon and coworkers[17] studied the effect of an alcohol extract of Bacopa monniera against nitrobenzene-induced liver damage. Adult male Wistar albino rats treated with nitrobenzene (50 mg/kg, PO) showed the following changes compared to the control group:

- Increased serum ALT, AST and ALP
- Increased liver LPO
- Decreased liver SOD, CAT and GPx
- Inflammation of the liver

Rats treated with nitrobenzene and BME (200 mg/kg/day, PO) showed a reversal of these changes. Nitrobenzene was administered on day 1. Treatment with BME started on day 2 and continued for 10 days. The authors concluded that "**the ethanolic extract of Bacopa monnieri plant produces good hepatoprotective activity.**"

Sumathi and Devaraj[28] investigated the effect of an ethanol extract of Bacopa monniera (BME) against morphine-induced liver and kidney toxicity. Adult male Wistar albino rats treated with morphine (10-160 mg/kg/day, PO) for 21 days showed increased serum marker enzymes, creatinine, uric acid and blood urea compared to the control group. They also showed damage to the liver and kidneys. Rats treated with morphine and BME (40 mg/kg/day, PO) for 21 days showed a reversal of these changes. The authors concluded that "**BME exerted a protective effect against morphine-induced liver and kidney toxicity.**"

Kannan and coworkers[29] examined the effect of an alcohol extract of Bacopa monniera (BME) on gentamicin (GM) induced nephrotoxicity in rats. Albino rats treated with GM (80 mg/kg/day, i.p.) for 15 days showed increased kidney LPO, serum urea, creatinine, uric acid and albumin, and decreased kidney antioxidants compared to the control group. Rats treated with GM and BME (100 or 200 mg/kg/day, PO) for 15 days showed a reversal of these changes. The authors concluded that the "**Bacopa monnieri extract attenuates renal injury in rats following gentamicin treatment, possibly by inhibiting lipid peroxidation and enhancing or maintaining the antioxidant potentials.**"

Bafna and Balaraman[30] studied the effect of DHC-1, a polyherbal formulation containing Bacopa monniera, on cisplatin-induced kidney damage in rats. Albino Wistar rats treated with cisplatin (3 mg/kg/day, i.p.) every 7 days for 28 days showed the following changes compared to the control group:

- Increased kidney LPO
- Increased serum creatinine, urea, uric acid and blood urea nitrogen
- Decreased kidney GSH, SOD, CAT, $Na^{+}K^{+}$ ATPase, Ca^{2+} ATPase and Mg^{2+} ATPase

Rats treated with cisplatin and DHC-1 (125-1000 mg/kg/day, PO) every 7 days for 28 days showed a reversal of these changes. The authors concluded that DHC-1 treatment offered significant protection from cisplatin-induced nephrotoxicity.

References

1 Cindy L Stanfield. Principles of Human Physiology. Pearson/Benjamin Cummings, 2011.

2 R K Sharma and Bhagwan Dash. Caraka Samhita (text with English translation and critical exposition based on Cakrapani Datta's Ayurveda Dipika) volume 4. Chowkhamba Sanskrit Series Office, Varanasi, India, Reprint 2007.

3 K R Srikantha Murthy. Illustrated Susruta Samhita. Vol III. Chaukhambha Orientalia, Varanasi, India, Reprint 2010.

4 K R Srikantha Murthy. Vagbhata's Astanga Hrdayam (text, English translation, notes, appendices and indices) volume 2. Chowkhamba Krishnadas Academy, Varanasi, India. Seventh edition, 2010.

5 Premalatha Balachandran, Rajgopal Govindarajan. "Hepatic disorders" in Scientific Basis for Ayurvedic Therapies. Edited by Lakshmi Chandra Mishra. CRC Press, Boca Raton, FL 2004.

6 M S Premila. Ayurvedic Herbs: a clinical guide to the healing plants of

traditional Indian medicine. The Haworth press Inc, Binghamton, NY, 2006.
7 Scott Treadway. An Ayurvedic herbal approach to a healthy liver. Clinical Nutrition Insights (1998) 6(16): 1-3.
8 G D Chaudhary, P Kamboj, I Singh, A N Kalia. Herbs as liver savers – a review. Indian Journal of Natural Products and Resources (2010) 1(4): 397-408.
9 A D Kshirsagar, R Mohite, A S Aggrawal, U R Suralkar. Hepatoprotective medicinal plants of Ayurveda – a review. Asian Journal of Pharmaceutical and Clinical Research (2011) 4(3): 1-8.
10 Manish V Patel, S N Gupta, Nimesh G Patel. Effects of Ayurvedic treatment on 100 patients of chronic renal failure (other than diabetic nephropathy). Ayu (2011) 32(4): 483-486.
11 Singh Karam, Verma Bhavna. Hepatoprotection through Ayurvedic herbs. International Journal of Ayurvedic and Herbal Medicine (2012) 2(5): 885-896.
12 P Bigoniya, C S Singh, A Shukla. A comparative review of different liver toxicants used in experimental pharmacology. International Journal of Pharmaceutical Sciences and Drug Research (2009) 1(3): 124-135.
13 Amy Schilling, Rebecca Corey, Mandy Leonard, Bijan Eghtesad. Acetaminophen: old drug, new warnings. Cleveland Clinic Journal of Medicine (2010) 77(1): 19-27.
14 Singh Robin, Kumar Sunil, Rana A C, Sharma Nidhi. Different models of hepatotoxicity and related liver diseases: a review. International Research Journal of Pharmacy (2012) 3(7): 86-95.
15 Femke Heindryckx, Isabelle Colle, Hans Van Vlierberghe. Experimental mouse models for hepatocellular carcinoma research. Int. J. Exp. Path. (2009) 90: 367-386.
16 US Environmental protection Agency. Toxicological review of nitrobenzene. http://www.epa.gov/iris/toxreviews/0079tr.pdf
17 B Rajalakshmy Menon, M A Rathi, L Thirumoorthi, V K Gopalakrishnan. Potential effect of Bacopa monnieri on nitrobenzene induced liver damage in rats. Indian Journal of Clinical Biochemistry (2010) 25(4): 401-404.
18 F Stain-Texier, P Sandouk, J M Scherrmann. Intestinal absorption and stability of morphine 6-glucuronide in different physiological compartments of the rat. Drug Metabolism and Disposition (1998) 26(5): 383-387.
19 Takashi Todaka, Takashi Ishida, Hideki Kita, Shizuo Narimatsu, Shigeru Yamano. Bioactivation of morphine in human liver: isolation and identification of morphinone a toxic metabolite. Biological and Pharmaceutical Bulletin (2005) 28(7): 1275-1280.
20 Amrit Pal Singh, Arunachalam Muthuraman, Amteshwar Singh Jaggi, Nirmal Singh, Kuldeep Grover, Ravi Dhawan. Animal models of acute renal failure. Pharmacological Reports (2012) 64: 31-44.
21 P Sangeetha, Charan D Swami, Sri K Janaki, D Sujatha, D Ranganayakul. Amelioration of gentamicin induced nephrotoxicity by egg in experimental animals. Journal of Pharmacy Research (2012) 5(5): 2636-2643.
22 Luis Alberto Batista Peres, Ademar Dantas da Cunha Júnior. Acute nephrotoxicity of cisplatin: molecular mechanisms. Jornal Brasileiro de

Nefrologia (2013) 35(4): 332-340.
23 T Sumathy, S Subramanian, S Govindasamy, K Balakrishna, G Veluchamy. Protective role of Bacopa monniera on morphine induced hepatotoxicity in rats. Phytotherapy Research (2001) 15: 643-645.
24 Tirtha Ghosh, Tapan Kumar Maity, Mrinmay Das, Anindya Bose, Deepak Kumar Dash. In vitro antioxidant and hepatoprotective activity of ethanolic extract of Bacopa monnieri Linn. aerial parts. Iranian Journal of Pharmacology and Therapeutics (2007) 6(1): 77-85.
25 T Sumathi, S Ramakrishnan. Hepatoprotective activity of Bacopa monniera on D-galactosamine induced hepatotoxicity in rats. Natural Product Sciences (2007) 13(3): 195-198.
26 T Sumathi, A Nongbri. Hepatoprotective effect of bacoside-A, a major constituent of Bacopa monniera Linn. Phytomedicine (2008) 15: 901-905.
27 Panneerselvam Janani, Kanakarajan Sivakumari, Chandrakesan Parthasarathy. Hepatoprotective activity of bacoside A against N-nitrosodiethylamine-induced liver toxicity. Cell Biology and Toxicology (2009) 25(5): 425-434.
28 T Sumathi, S Niranjali Devaraj. Effect of Bacopa monniera on liver and kidney toxicity in chronic use of opioids. Phytomedicine (2009) 16: 897-903.
29 N Ramesh Kannan, A Sudha, A Manimaran, D Saravanan, E Natarajan. Beneficial effect of Bacopa monnieri extract on gentamicin induced nephrotoxicity and oxidative stress in albino rats. International Journal of Pharmacy and Pharmaceutical Sciences (2011) 3(suppl 5): 144-148.
30 P A Bafna, R Balaraman. Antioxidant activity of DHC-1, an herbal formulation, in experimentally-induced cardiac and renal damage. Phytotherapy Research (2005) 19: 216-221.

17 – Cardioprotective Activity

17.1 – General

Cardiovascular disease (CVD) is a group of disorders of the heart and blood vessels. CVD is the leading cause of morbidity and mortality worldwide, with an estimated 17.3 million deaths in 2008[1]. Behavioral risk factors include unhealthy diet, lack of physical activity, tobacco use and excessive alcohol. Treatment of CVD includes lifestyle changes, medications, surgery and other medical procedures.

17.2 – Ayurveda and Heart Disease

In Ayurveda, heart disease is known as Hridaya Roga, and has been described in classic texts[2-4]. There are five types of heart disease in Ayurveda: vataja, pittaja, kaphaja, tridoshaja and karmija (due to infections). Ayurveda utilizes a number of plant-based drugs in the treatment of heart disease[5-8].

17.3 – Experimental Evidence

Nandev and coworkers[9] investigated the effect of a hydroalcoholic extract of Bacopa monniera (BM) on isoproterenol (ISP) induced myocardial necrosis in rats. Male Wistar albino rats treated with the vehicle for 30 days and administered with ISP (85 mg/kg, SC) on days 29 and 30 showed increased myocardial LPO and decreased LDH, CK-MB, SOD, CAT, GSH and GPx compared to the control group. They also showed myocardial damage. Rats treated with BM (50-200 mg/kg/day, PO) for 30 days and injected with ISP on days 29 and 30 showed a reversal of these changes. The authors concluded that the hydroalcoholic extract of Bacopa monniera **"provides significant cardioprotection against ISP-induced exogenous stress in rats."**

Mohanty and coworkers[10] examined the effect of a hydroalcoholic lyophilized extract of Bacopa monniera (BM) against ISP-induced myocardial injury. Adult male Wistar rats treated with the vehicle for 21 days and injected with ISP (85 mg/kg, SC) on days 20 and 21 showed myonecrosis, increased myocardial LPO and decreased GSH, SOD, and creatine phosphokinase (CPK) compared to the control group. Rats treated with BM (25-150 mg/kg/day, PO) for 21 days and injected with ISP on days 20 and 21 showed a reversal of these changes. The investigators concluded that **"BM offered significant protection against ISP induced myocardial necrosis through a unique property of enhancement of endogenous antioxidants without producing any cytotoxic effects."**

In a subsequent investigation, Mohanty and coworkers[11] demonstrated the cardioprotective effect of a Bacopa monniera extract (BM) using the Langendorff model. Hearts from rats treated with saline for 21 days and subjected to ischaemia-reperfusion (IR) showed the following changes compared to the control group:

- Depression in heart rate
- Decreased endogenous antioxidants and CPK
- Increased LPO
- Increased Bax expression and decreased Bcl-2 expression
- Strong Hsp72 expression
- Necrosis, edema and inflammation

Hearts from rats treated with BM (75 mg/kg/day, PO) and subjected to IR showed a reversal of these changes. The cardioprotective effect of BM was attributed to its antioxidant and apoptotic properties. The investigators concluded that **"the study provides scientific basis for the putative therapeutic effect of B. monniera in ischaemic heart disease."**

Bafna and Balaraman[12] studied the effect of DHC-1, a polyherbal formulation containing Bacopa monniera, on ISP-induced cardiac injury in rats. Albino Wistar rats treated with the vehicle for 30 days and injected with ISP (25 mg/kg, SC) on days 30 and 31 showed the following changes compared to the control group:

- Increased serum CK, LDH, uric acid, GOT and heart LPO
- Decreased heart GSH, CAT, $Na^{+}K^{+}$ ATPase, Ca^{2+} ATPase and Mg^{2+} ATPase

Rats treated with DHC-1 (125-1000 mg/kg/day, PO) for 30 days and injected with ISP on days 30 and 31 showed a reversal of these changes.

References

1 World Health Organization. Cardiovascular disease (CVDS): Fact Sheet No. 317. March 2013.

2 R K Sharma and Bhagwan Dash. Caraka Samhita (text with English translation and critical exposition based on Cakrapani Datta's Ayurveda Dipika) volume 4. Chowkhamba Sanskrit Series Office, Varanasi, India, Reprint 2007

3 K R Srikantha Murthy. Illustrated Susruta Samhita, Vol III. Chaukhambha Orientalia, Varanasi, India. Fourth edition 2010.

4 K R Srikantha Murthy. Vagbhata's Astanga Hrdayam (text, English translation, notes, appendices and indices) volume 1. Chowkhamba Krishnadas Academy, Varanasi, India. Seventh edition, 2010.

5 Karunkaran Gauthaman, Lakshmi Chandra Mishra. "Ischemic heart disease" in Scientific Basis for Ayurvedic Therapies. Edited by Lakshmi Chandra Mishra. CRC Press, Boca Raton, FL, 2004.

6 M S Premila. Ayurvedic Herbs: a clinical guide to the healing plants of traditional Indian medicine. The Haworth press Inc, Binghamton, NY, 2006.

7 P D Lokhande, S C Jagdale, A R Chabukswar. Natural remedies for heart diseases. Indian Journal of Traditional Knowledge (2006) 5(3): 420-427.

8 Ipseeta Ray Mohanty, Suresh Kumar Gupta, Nimain Mohanty, Daniel Joseph, Yeshwant Deshmukh. The beneficial effects of herbs in cardiovascular diseases. Global Journal of Medical Research (2012) 12(4): 38-58.

9 Mukesh Nandave, Shreesh K Ojha, Sujata Joshi, Santosh Kumari, Dharamvir S Arya. Cardioprotective effect of Bacopa monniera against isoproterenol-induced myocardial necrosis in rats. International Journal of Pharmacology (2007) 3(5): 385-392.

10 Ipseeta Ray Mohanty, Ujjwala Maheswari, Daniel Joseph, Vijay Moghe. Bacopa monniera augments endogenous antioxidants and attenuates myocardial injury. International Journal of Integrative Biology (2009) 7: 73-79.

11 Ipseeta Ray Mohanty, Ujjwala Maheswari, Daniel Joseph, Yeshwant Deshmukh. Bacopa monniera protects rat heart against ischaemia-reperfusion injury: role of key apoptotic regulatory proteins and enzymes. Journal of Pharmacy and Pharmacology (2010) 62: 1175-1184.

12 P A Bafna, R Balaraman. Antioxidant activity of DHC-1, an herbal formulation, in experimentally induced cardiac and renal damage. Phytotherapy Research (2005) 19: 216-221.

18 – Effect on Cancer

18.1 – General

In spite of decades of relentless efforts to find a cure for cancer, it is still one of the most dreadful maladies. An estimated 12.7 million cases of cancer and 7.6 million cancer deaths occurred in 2008[1].

Cancer is not just one disease. It is a group of diseases characterized by the uncontrolled growth and spread of abnormal cells. Most cancers are named for the organ or type of cell that is initially affected[2]. Normal cells follow an orderly path of growth, division and death, but this process gets disturbed sometimes (e.g. by mutations in the DNA of a cell). When this happens, cells do not die when they should (apoptosis) and new cells do not form as they should. The extra cells may form a mass of tissue called a tumor, which can be benign (noncancerous) or malignant (cancerous). Benign tumors tend to grow slowly and do not spread. Cells in malignant tumors invade and destroy nearby normal tissues, and spread throughout the body (metastasis).

The causes of cancer are many and include individual lifestyle, environment and family history[3]. Treatment depends on the type and stage of cancer, age, health status and other factors. Treatments include surgery, radiation and chemotherapy.

18.2 – Ayurveda and Cancer

Ancient Ayurvedic texts[4-6] mention diseases with clinical features similar to cancer such as Apache, Gulma, Granthi and Arbuda. Tumors are classified as follows: vataja arbuda, pittaja arbuda, raktaja arbuda, mamsaja arbuda and medaja arbuda[7]. Treatment is mainly based on shodhana and shamana procedures. Various plant-based drugs and formulations have been mentioned for the management of cancer. Recently, a number of articles on the Ayurvedic perspective on cancer have appeared[7-13].

18.3 – Experimental Evidence

The cytotoxicity of different extracts of Bacopa monniera (BM) has been evaluated by a number of researchers[14-19] using the brine shrimp lethality test. This test is well correlated with antitumor activity[20]. Some published results are summarized below (Table 18.1):

Extracts/Compounds	IC_{50}/LC_{50} Values		Ref
Bacopa monniera (leaf) was extracted successively with petroleum ether, chloroform, ethanol and water. A saponin rich fraction (SRF) was also prepared. Bacoside A was isolated from the SRF.		LC_{50} (μg/mL)	14
	Bacoside A	38.3	
	SRF	95.4	
	Ethanol extract	295.5	
Bacopa monniera was extracted with 70% methanol. The methanol extract and a number of other compounds isolated from Bacopa monniera were tested. Compounds with IC_{50} values less than 100 mg/mL are shown here.		IC_{50} (μg/mL)	15
	Bacopasaponin C	3.9	
	Bacoside A	29	
	Bacopaside II	32.5	
	Bacopaside X	36.1	
	Bacopaside B	65	
	Methanol extract	70	
	Bacopaside I	75	
Aqueous extract	LC_{50} = 90 μg/mL		16
Bacopa monniera (aerial parts) was extracted with methanol. The extract was suspended in water and then successively partitioned with CH_2Cl_2, EtOAc and n-BuOH.		LC_{50} (μg/mL)	17
	CH_2Cl_2 fraction	19.02	
	Methanol extract	34.92	
	EtOAc fraction	45.32	
	n-BuOH fraction	84.65	
95% ethanol extract	LC_{50} = 40 μg/mL		18
80% methanol extract (leaves)	LC_{50} = 26.30 μg/mL		19

Table 18.1: Brine shrimp lethality bioassays of BM

Rohini and coworkers[21] evaluated the antioxidant and tumor-inhibiting effects of an alcohol extract of Bacopa monniera (BM) in fibrosarcoma-bearing rats. Fibrosarcoma was induced in male albino rats with 3-methylcholanthrene. Serially transplanted animals were maintained by subcutaneous injections of the tumor tissue suspended in saline in the flank area of the rats. On the 10th day after tumor tissue injection, the fibrosarcoma-bearing (FB) rats were treated with or without BM (20 mg/kg/day, SC) for 30 days. Normal rats were also studied for comparison. FB rats not treated with BM showed increased LPO and SOD, CAT, GSH and GPx (liver and kidney) as well as increased serum markers LDH, ALT and sialic acid compared to untreated normal rats. FB rats treated with BM showed a reversal of these changes. The authors concluded that "**B. monniera extract promotes the antioxidant status, reduces the rate of lipid peroxidation and the markers of tumor progression in the fibrosarcoma bearing rats.**"

In a subsequent investigation, Rohini[22] showed the tumor-inhibiting effect of an ethanol extract of Bacopa monniera (BM) in fibrosarcoma-bearing (FB) rats. FB rats treated with BM (20 mg/kg/day, SC) for 30 days showed the following changes compared to untreated FB rats:

- Increased survival time
- Decreased tumor rate
- Decreased serum γGT, cathespin–D, ceruloplasmin and circulating immune complexes (CIC)

A histological section of tumor tissues taken from the right flank of FB rats treated with BM showed small clusters of tumor cells. Tumor tissues from untreated FB rats showed a well-differentiated fibrosarcoma with a typical herringbone pattern. The author concluded that "**the ethanolic extract of B. monniera inhibits tumor progression in fibrosarcoma bearing rats.**"

Rohini and Shyamala Devi[23] investigated the effect of an ethanol extract of Bacopa monniera (BM) on apoptosis in murine sarcoma cells (S-180). Cells treated with BM (50-550 mg/mL) showed mortality in a dose- and time-dependent manner. Maximum cytotoxicity was observed at a concentration of 550 mg/mL at 48 h. Electron microscopy and an Annexin V-FITC assay of S-180 cells treated with BM (450 or 550 mg/mL) showed apoptosis. The authors concluded that "**BM induces cell death by apoptosis in S-180 cells.**"

Ghosh and coworkers[24] examined the effect of stigmasterol isolated from Bacopa monniera against Ehrlich ascites carcinoma (EAC) in mice. Swiss albino mice were injected with EAC cells in ice cold saline. They were treated with the vehicle, stigmasterol (5 or 10 mg/kg/day, i.p.) or 5-fluorouracil (20 mg/kg/day, i.p.) for 7 days. EAC mice treated with stigmasterol or 5-fluorouracil showed the following changes compared to EAC mice treated with the vehicle:

- Increased mean survival time and decreased tumor weight

- Increased hemoglobin (Hb) content, RBC, and platelet count (PLC), and decreased WBC compared to vehicle-treated EAC mice.
- Increased monocytes and lymphocytes, and decreased neutrophils in a differential count of WBC
- Decreased LPO and increased GSH, SOD and CAT in liver tissues
- Decreased LDH activity in ascites fluid
- Less liver tissue damage

The investigators stated that "**stigmasterol might be a potent lead molecule in search of a nontoxic, plant origin anti cancer agent.**"

Mastan and coworkers[25] examined the chemoprotective effect of an ethanol extract of Bacopa monniera (BM) on the biochemical changes in chick embryos induced by cytarabine, also known as cytosine arabinoside (CA). CA is an effective anticancer drug, but it causes adverse biochemical changes. Freshly laid Bobcock strain fertilized eggs (zero days old) were divided into three groups and treated as follows:

Group	Treatment
1	Saline (control)
2	CA (3 mg) on day 15
3	BM (2, 4 or 6 mg) on day 12 + CA (3 mg) on day 15

The embryos were exposed 24 hours after CA administration. Amniotic fluid and tissues of the liver, heart and brain were collected for biochemical analysis. Major findings from this study are presented below (Table 18.2):

Assay	CA (2) compared to Control (1)	BM + CA (3) compared to CA (2)
ALP, AST, ALT, LDH, MDH (amniotic fluid)	Increased	Decreased
ALP, AST, ALT, LDH, MDH (liver)	Increased	Decreased
AST, ALT, LDH, MDH (heart)	Increased	Decreased

Table 18.2: Effects of BM on cytarbine-induced biochemical changes in chick embryos

Peng and coworkers[26] evaluated the antitumor activity (both in vitro and in vivo) of a methanol extract of Bacopa monniera (whole plant) and fractions of the methanol extract obtained by successive fractionation with petroleum ether, $CHCl_3$, EtOAc and n-BuOH. The cytotoxic activity of the methanol extract and its fractions were tested (in vitro) against human cancer cell lines. Major findings from this study are summarized below:

- The EtOAc fraction showed no cytotoxicity against any of the cell lines tested, and the petroleum ether fraction showed minimal cytotoxicity.
- The methanol extract was cytotoxic to all tested tumor lines.
- The $CHCl_3$ fraction was cytotoxic to the human cancer cell lines MDA-MB-231, SHG-40 and HCT-8.
- The n-BuOH fraction showed the highest overall cytotoxicity. Four compounds from the n-BuOH fraction were isolated and tested, two of which (bacopaside II and bacopasaponin C) were not very potent. The other two compounds, bacopaside E and bacopaside VII, showed cytotoxicity against all cell lines tested.

The in vivo study showed that bacoside E and bacopaside VII inhibited sarcoma S180 tumor growth in mice.

Janani and coworkers[27] evaluated the chemopreventive effect of bacoside A (BA) against DEN-induced hepatocarcinogenesis in rats. Adult male Wistar albino rats treated with DEN (0.01%) in drinking water for 16 weeks showed the following changes compared to the control group:

- Increased relative liver weight
- 100% liver tumor nodule incidence
- Increased tumor markers α-feto proteins, carcinoembryonic antigen and 5'-nucleotidase
- Increased serum marker enzymes
- Decreased endogenous antioxidants in hemolysate and liver

Rats treated with DEN and BA (15 mg/kg/day, PO) for 16 weeks showed a reversal of these changes. Histopathological and ultrastructural studies of liver tissues of DEN-treated rats showed loss of architecture and other alterations indicative of hepatocarcinogenesis. Rats treated with DEN and BA showed less loss of architecture and other alterations. The investigators suggested that "**bacoside A may be used as an effective drug for cancer treatment.**"

Janani and coworkers[28] investigated the effect of bacoside A (BA) on the activities and expressions of matrix metalloproteinase 2 and 9 (MMP-2 and MMP-9) in DEN-induced hepatocellular carcinoma. MMP-2 and MMP-9 have been implicated in tumor metastasis. The experimental design was similar to the one described previously[27]. Rats treated with BM + DEN showed decreased activities of MMP-2, MMP-9 as well as MMP-2 and MMP-9 expressions compared to the DEN-only group. The authors concluded that **"BA has a potent anti-metastatic effect against DEN-induced hepatocellular carcinoma in rats by reducing the activities and expression of MMP-2 and MMP-9."**

Kalyani and coworkers[29] evaluated the cytotoxic effect of various extracts of Bacopa monniera in mouse mammary carcinoma cells. Swiss albino mice (6-8 weeks old) were injected with Ehrlich ascites tumor (EAT) cells. After 6 days, these EAT-bearing mice were divided into groups and treated with the extracts individually (500 mg/day, i.p.) until the 12th day. Untreated EAT-bearing mice served as the control group. The aqueous extract (BMWE) was found to be the most effective treatment, and its results are summarized below:

- BMWE-treated EAT-bearing mice survived longer and showed less body weight gain, lower EAT cell counts and decreased ascite fluid volume compared to the control group.
- BMWE-treated EAT-bearing mice showed a decrease in peritoneal angiogenesis compared to the control group. Histological examination of the peritoneal section of BMWE-treated EAT-bearing mice showed decreased microvessel density (MVD) compared to the control group. Ascites from BMWE-treated EAT-bearing mice showed decreased vascular endothelial growth factor, a signal protein that stimulates angiogenesis.
- EAT cells from BMWE-treated EAT-bearing mice showed apoptotic morphological characteristics and DNA fragmentation. Cytosolic extracts showed endonuclease activity on salmon sperm DNA.

An in vitro study was done using EAT cells. The results are summarized below:

- In the presence of a specific caspase 3 inhibitor, treatment of EAT cells with BMWE showed inhibition of DNA fragmentation.
- Nuclear extracts of BMWE-treated EAT cells degraded plasmid DNA. Caspase-activated DNase (CAD) was detected in the nuclear extract, indicating the involvement of CAD in oligonucleosomal DNA fragmentation.

- BMWE-treated EAT cells showed decreased Bcl-2 (an anti-apoptotic gene) expression and increased Bax (a pro-apoptotic gene) expression.
- BMWE inhibited the proliferation of EAT cells.

The authors stated that **"BMWE was able to induce apoptosis in EAT cells via Bax-related caspase-3 activation. This may provide experimental data for the further clinical use of BMWE in cancer."**

Multiple studies[30,31] have reported that Bacopa monniera reduced papilloma formation in Swiss albino mice initiated by 7,12-dimethylbenz(a)anthracene (DMBA) and promoted with croton oil.

References

1 A Jemal, F Bray, M M Center, J Ferlay, E Ward, D Forman. Global Cancer Statistics. CA Cancer J Clin (2011) 61(2): 69-90.
2 National Cancer Institute. What is cancer? http://www.cancer.gov/cancertopics/cancerlibrary/what-is-cancer
3 World Health Organization. Cancer: fact sheet No. 297. January 2013.
4 R K Sharma and Bhagwan Dash. Caraka Samhita (text with English translation and critical exposition based on Cakrapani Datta's Ayurveda Dipika) Volume 4. Chowkhamba Sanskrit Series Office, Varanasi, India, Reprint 2007.
5 K R Srikantha Murthy. Illustrated Susruta Samhita. Vol II. Chaukhambha Orientalia, Varanasi, India, Reprint 2010.
6 K R Srikantha Murthy. Vagbhata's Astanga Hrdayam (text, English translation, notes, appendices and indices). Chowkhamba Krishnadas Academy, Varanasi, India. Seventh edition, 2010.
7 Manoranjan Sahu, Lakshmi Chandra Mishra. "Benign growths, cysts, and malignant tumors" in Scientific Basis for Ayurvedic Therapies. Edited by Lakshmi Chandra Mishra. CRC Press, Boca Raton, FL, 2004.
8 Premalatha Balachandran, Rajgopal Govindarajan. Cancer – an Ayurvedic perspective. Pharmacological Research (2005) 51: 19-30.
9 Avnish K Upadhyay, Arvind Kumar, Hari S Mishra. An integrated approach to combat cancer (neoplasm): in perspective of Ayurveda. Indian Journal of Ancient Medicine and Yoga (2009) 2(1): 3-8.
10 Ashok D B Vaidya, Ashok J Amonkar, Narendra S Bhatt, Purvish M Parikh. "Complimentary and alternative medicine for cancer care in India: basic and clinical perspective" in Alternative and Complementary Therapies for Cancer. Edited by Moulay Alaoui-Jamali. Springer, New York, 2010.
11 Dipal Patel, Ahamed Noor Mansori. Cancer – an Ayurvedic perspective. IJARPB (2012) 2(2): 179-195.
12 V N Sumantran, G Tillu. Cancer, inflammation and insights from Ayurveda. eCAM (2012). doi:10.1155/2012/306346
13 Subhash Singh, Shiv Kumar Singh, Narendra Kumar Singh. Cancer in

Ayurveda. Int. Journal of Basic and Applied Medical Sciences (2012) 2(3): 162-165.

14 P D'Souza, M Deepak, P Rani, S Kadamboor, A Mathew, A P Chandrashekar, A Agarwal. Brine shrimp lethality assay of Bacopa monnieri. Phytother Res (2002) 16(2): 197-198.

15 Chillara Sivaramakrishna, Chirravuri V Rao, Golakoti Trimurtulu, Mulabagal Vanisree, Gottumukkala V Subbaraju. Triterpenoid glycosides from Bacopa monnieri. Phytochemistry (2005) 66(23): 2719-2728.

16 Alluri V Krishnaraju, Tayi V N Rao, Dodda Sundararaju, Mulabagal Vanisree, Hsin-Sheng Tsay, Gottumukkala V Subbaraju. Biological screening of medicinal plants collected from eastern Ghats of India using Artemia salina (brine shrimp test). Int J Appl Sci Eng (2006) 4(2): 115-125.

17 M B Alam, M S Hossain, M Asadujjaman, M M Islam, M E H Mazumder, M E Haque. Peroxynitrite scavenging and toxicity potential of different fractions of the aerial parts of Bacopa monniera Linn. International Journal of Pharmaceutical Sciences and Drug Research (2010) 1(10): 78-83.

18 H Hossain, Md S I Howlader, S K Dey, A Hira, A Ahmed. Evaluation of analgesic, antidiarrhoeal and cytotoxic activities of ethanolic extract of Bacopa monnieri (L). Brit J Pharm Res (2012) 2(3): 188-196.

19 Siraj Md Afjalus, Newton Chakma, Mahmudur Rahman, Malik Salahuddin, Sadhu Samir Kumar. Assessment of analgesic, antidiarrhoeal and cytotoxic activity of ethanolic extract of the whole plant of Bacopa monnieri Linn. International Research Journal of Pharmacy (2012) 3(10): 98-101.

20 T R Prashith Kekuda, H L Raghavendra, K S Surabhi, H R Preethi, S P Swarnalatha. Cytotoxic activity of methanol extract of Abrus pulchellus Wall (Fabaceae) leaves. Biomedicine (2010) 30(3): 377-379.

21 G Rohini, K E Sabitha, C S Shyamala Devi. Bacopa monniera Linn. extract modulates antioxidant and marker enzyme status in fibrosarcoma bearing rats. Indian Journal of Experimental Biology (2004) 42: 776-780.

22 G Rohini. Bacopa monniera extract inhibits tumor promotion in fibrosarcoma bearing rats. Journal of Natural Remedies (2008) 8(1): 101-108.

23 G Rohini, C S Shyamala Devi. Bacopa monniera extract induces apoptosis in murine sarcoma cells (S-180). Phytotherapy Research (2008) 22: 1595-1598.

24 T Ghosh, T K Maity, J Singh. Evaluation of antitumor activity of stigmasterol, a constituent isolated from Bacopa monnieri Linn aerial parts against ehrlich ascites carcinoma in mice. Orient Pharm Exp Med (2011) 11: 41-49.

25 M Mastan, U V Prasad, P R Parthasarathy. Protective effect of Bacopa monniera L. on cytarabine induced biochemical changes in chick Embryo. Indian Journal of Clinical Biochemistry (2007) 22(1): 122-127.

26 Ling Peng, Yun Zhou, De Yun Kong, Wei Dong Zhang. Antitumor activities of dammarane triterpene saponins from Bacopa monniera. Phytotherapy Research (2010) 24: 864-868.

27 P Janani, K Sivakumari, A Geetha, B Ravisankar, C Parthasarathy. Chemopreventive effect of bacoside A on N-nitrosodiethylamine-induced hepatocarcinogenesis in rats. J Cancer Res Clini Oncol (2010) 136: 759-770.

28 P Janani, K Sivakumari, A Geetha, S Yuvaraj, C Parthasarathy. Bacoside A downregulates matrix metalloproteinases 2 and 9 in DEN-induced

hepatocellular carcinoma. Cell Biochemistry and Function (2010) 28: 164-169.

29 M I Kalyani, S M Lingaraju, B P Salimath. A pro-apoptotic 15-kDa protein from Bacopa monnieri activates caspase-3 and downregulates Bcl-2 gene expression in mouse mammary carcinoma cells. J. Nat Med (2013) 67: 123-126.

30 N Gaidhani, V Lokhande, K Girhepunje, R Pal. Effect of Becopa monnieri on DMBA-induced Swiss Albino mice skin tumorigenesis: a preliminary study. Asian Journal of Pharmaceutical Education and Research (2012) 1(1): 90-102.

31 Shiki Vishnoi, R C Agarwal. Chemopreventive action of Bacopa monnieri (Brahmi) hydromethanolic extract of DMBA-induced skin carcinogenesis in Swiss albino mice. J Pharmacogn Phytochem (2013) 2(2): 197-202.

19 – Antimicrobial Activity

19.1 – General

Since the introduction of penicillin in the early 1940s, antibiotics have played a vital role in the fight against infectious diseases. These 'miracle' drugs have saved countless lives all over the world. They are essential in controlling a number of bacterial infections. However, bacteria and other microbes are highly resilient and capable of developing resistance to antibiotics. During the past few decades, antibiotics have been used indiscriminately and inappropriately. If the misuse and overuse of antibiotics continues, there is the risk of having no defense against these deadly microbes[1]. It is critical to explore alternative strategies to treat microbial infection, and save the magic bullet (antibiotics) as a last resort.

19.2 – Ayurveda and Infectious Diseases

Microorganisms and infectious diseases were known in the early days of Ayurveda. In the Atharvaveda, microorganisms and infectious diseases are referred to as Krimi and Krimi Rogas, respectively[2]. Major works on Ayurveda have described these in detail[3-5]. Charaka[3] mentions twenty types of pathogenic krimis, which are classified into four groups: Purisaja (born of feces), Slesmaja (born of phlegm), Sonitaja (born of blood) and Malaja (born of external excreta). Charaka discusses three main approaches for treating krimi rogas: Apakarshana (removal of krimis), Prakriti Vighata (stopping the growth of krimis by creating unfavorable conditions for growth) and Vidana Parivarjana (avoidance of causative factors). A number of papers on the antibacterial properties of plants used in the treatment of krimi rogas have recently been published[6-15].

19.3 – Experimental Evidence

Chaudhari and coworkers[16] investigated the antifungal activity of betulinic acid isolated from Bacopa monniera against the fungi Alternaria alternata and Fusarium fusiformis. The fungi were isolated from the diseased parts of some medicinal and aromatic plants. Betulinic acid inhibited A. alternata (IC_{50} = 2.3 μg/mL) and did not show any effect against F. Fusiformis.

Ghosh and coworkers[17] found that an ethanol extract of Bacopa monniera (aerial parts) was effective against a number of gram-positive bacteria, gram-negative bacteria, and fungi. Ciprofloxacin (5 mg/mL) and clotrimazole (25 mg/mL) were used as the reference standards for antibacterial and antifungal studies, respectively. Antimicrobial activity was evaluated by determining the minimum inhibitory concentration (broth dilution method) and zone of inhibition (agar disc diffusion method). The minimum inhibitory concentration study showed that the extract (50-400 mg/mL) was effective against all of the tested microorganisms. In the zone inhibition study, the extract (2-10 mg/mL) was effective in a dose-dependent manner, comparable to the reference standards. The extract was more effective against gram-positive bacteria than gram-negative bacteria.

In a subsequent study, Ghosh and coworkers[18] showed the antimicrobial activity of ethyl acetate and n-butanol fractions of an ethanol extract of Bacopa monniera (aerial parts) against the microorganisms in the previous study. The ethyl acetate fraction was found to be more effective than the n-butanol fraction.

Mandal and coworkers[19] reported the antibacterial activity of an ethanol extract of Bacopa monniera (leaf) against Salmonella enterica serovar typhi, a causal organism of typhoid fever. The extract showed a 10-18 mm zone diameter of inhibition (ZDI) around the wells, indicating antibacterial activity. The minimum inhibitory concentration study showed antibacterial activity of the extract (50-600 μg/mL). A bacterial killing study was also conducted. The extract (500 μg/mL) reduced cells from 50,000 cfu/mL to 48 cfu/mL.

Sampath Kumar and coworkers[20] examined the antimicrobial activity of different extracts of Bacopa monniera against Staphylococcus aureus, Proteus vulgaris, Candida albicans, and Aspergillus niger. Ethanolic, diethyl ether, ethyl acetate and water extracts of Bacopa monniera were used. The aqueous extract (100-300 μg/mL) did not show antimicrobial activity against any of the microorganisms tested. The other extracts showed antimicrobial activity against all microorganisms tested. At the extract concentration of 300 μg/mL, antimicrobial activity decreased in the following order:

Microorganism	Order of antimicrobial activity
S. aureus	Diethyl ether > Ethanol > Ethyl acetate
P. vulgaris	Ethyl acetate > Diethyl ether > Ethanol
C. albicans	Ethanol > Diethyl ether > Ethyl acetate
A. niger	Ethanol > Diethyl ether > Ethyl acetate

Sengupta and coworkers[21] screened an ethanol extract of Bacopa monniera leaves and young shoot tips (BME) for antifungal activity against sixteen fungal strains. The extract was found to have antifungal activity against Curvularia lunata (ZDI=18 mm), Rhizoctonia solani (ZDI=18 mm), Alternaria brassicicola (ZDI=16 mm), and Acremonium kiliense (ZDI=15 mm).

In vivo antifungal activity of the extract against Rhizoctonia solani was also investigated. R. solani causes diseases in rice and other plants. A field trial with rice seeds was conducted using the seed treatment and foliar spray methods. BME showed antifungal activity in both methods. The seed treatment method was more effective.

Rajashekharappa and coworkers[22] screened a methanol extract of Bacopa monniera and bacoside A for their antibacterial activity against pathogenic strains belonging to gram-negative Pseudomonas aeruginosa and Klebsiella pneumoniae, and gram-positive Staphylococcus aureus. The bacteria strains were collected from infected patients not treated with antibiotics. Ciprofloxacin (0.5 mg/mL) was used as the reference standard. The results are summarized below:

- The methanol extract (1 mg/mL) exhibited strong antimicrobial activity against S. aureus strains (ZDI=19.33-22.0 mm), and moderate activity against K. pneumnoniae (ZDI=13.0-15.0 mm) and P. aeruginosa (ZDI=11.67-13.33 mm).
- Bacoside A also showed strong activity against S. aureus strains (ZDI=20.32-21.33 mm), and moderate activity against K. pneumoniae (ZDI=14.23-16.18 mm) and P. aeruginosa (ZDI=13.08-14.08 mm).
- Ciprofloxacin showed strong activity against S. aureus (ZDI=19.0-22.85 mm), K. pneumoniae (ZDI=17.0-20.63 mm) and P. aeruginosa (ZDI=16.77-20.58 mm).

Khan and coworkers[23] evaluated the antibacterial activity of aqueous and methanol extracts of Bacopa monniera as well a number of methanol extract fractions against seven gram-positive and eleven gram-negative species of bacteria. Fractions were prepared by sequential extraction of the methanol extract with petroleum ether, benzene and ethyl acetate. The methanol extract and ethyl acetate fractions were most effective, followed by the aqueous extract, benzene fraction and petroleum ether fraction. The methanol extract and ethyl acetate fraction exhibited antibacterial activity against fifteen bacterial species, including all of the gram-positive bacteria. The aqueous extract was effective against all of the gram-positive bacteria and five of the gram-negative bacteria.

Ayyappan and coworkers[24] reported the antibacterial activity of aqueous and ethanol extracts of Bacopa monniera (leaf) against some common bacterial strains from humans. The ethanol extract was found to be more effective than the aqueous extract.

Mathur and coworkers[25] evaluated the antimicrobial activity of aqueous, hexane, methanol and petroleum ether extracts of Bacopa monniera against a number of bacteria and fungi. Chloramphenicol and fluconazole were used as the antibacterial and antifungal reference standards, respectively. The methanol extract showed the highest antimicrobial activity among the extracts, and its effects were comparable to both chloramphenicol and fluconazole. The petroleum ether and hexane extracts showed somewhat lower antimicrobial activity. The aqueous extract showed no antimicrobial activity against any of the microorganisms tested.

Alam and coworkers[26] evaluated the antimicrobial activity of a methanol extract of Bacopa monniera (leaf callus) against a number of bacteria and fungi. Ciprofloxacin and griseofulvin were used as the antibacterial and antifungal reference standards, respectively. The extract exhibited antibacterial and antifungal activity against all of the microorganisms tested. Its effects were comparable to the reference standards.

Azad and coworkers[27] showed the antimicrobial activity of an ether extract of Bacopa monniera (root, bark and stem bark) against the microorganisms Salmonella typhi (ZDI=21 mm), Staphylococcus aureus (ZDI=19 mm), Bacillus cereus (ZDI=18 mm) and Candida albicans (ZDI=16 mm).

Kalaivani and coworkers[28] evaluated the antibacterial activity of several extracts of Bacopa monniera against a number of gram-positive and gram-negative bacteria. The extracts were prepared by sequential extraction of air-dried aerial parts of Bacopa monniera with petroleum ether, benzene, DCM, chloroform, ethanol and water. The results are summarized below:

- The ethanol and DCM extracts were more effective than the other extracts. The ethanol extract showed antibacterial activity against Streptococcus pneumonia, Enterococcus faecalis, Proteus mirabilis and Klebsiella pneumoniae.

- The benzene and chloroform extracts showed low activity against gram-positive bacteria and no activity against gram-negative bacteria.
- The aqueous extract was moderately active.
- The petroluem ether extract was not effective against any of the organisms tested.

Vetriselvan and coworkers[29] demonstrated the antibacterial activity of Bacopa monniera and a polyherbal formulation containing equal amounts of Withania somnifera, Bacopa monniera and Cinnamomum zeylanicum against Klesiella aerogenes, Pseudomonas aeruginosa and Escherichia coli. The ZDI values for Bacopa monniera were 16 mm (K. aerogenes), 16 mm (P. aeruginosa) and 17 mm (E. coli). For the polyherbal formulation, ZDI values were 19 mm (K. aerogenes), 17 mm (P. aeruginosa) and 16 mm (E. coli).

Udgire and Pathade[30] evaluated the antifungal activity of different extracts of the leaves and whole plant of Bacopa monniera against Aspergillus niger ATCC 16404, Candida albicans ATCC 10231 and Malassezia furfur MTCC 1765. The methanol and methanol-ethanol extracts of both leaves and whole plant were more potent than the other extracts against all of the pathogens. The methanol and methanol-ethanol extracts were analyzed by GC-MS and 19 compounds were identified. The major constituent of the methanol extract was identified as oxirane, a precursor for the preparation of triazole antifungal agents.

References

1 Scott Treadway. Exploring the universe of Ayurvedic botanicals to manage bacterial infections. Clinical Nutrition Insights (1998) 6(17): 1-3.

2 G S Lavekar, Alka Babbar. "Antimicrobial activities of some Ayurvedic plant drugs: an appraisal of evidence based researches" in Microbes: Health and Environment. Edited by Ashok K. Chauhan and Ajit Varma. I. K. International Publishing House Pvt Ltd, New Delhi, 2006.

3 R K Sharma and Bhagwan Dash. Caraka Samhita (text with English translation and critical exposition based on Cakrapani Datta's Ayurveda Dipika) volume 2. Chowkhamba Sanskrit Series Office, Varanasi, India, Reprint 2007.

4 K R Srikantha Murthy. Vagbhata's Astanga Hrdayam (text, English translation, notes, appendices and indices) volume 2. Chowkhamba Krishnadas Academy, Varanasi, India. Seventh edition, 2010.

5 K R Srikantha Murthy. Bhavaprakasa of Bhavamisra (text, English translation, notes, appendices and index) volume 2. Chowkhamba Krishnadas Academy, Varanasi, Fourth Edition 2008.

6 Mahendra K Rai, Nandkishore J Chickhale, Manjusha J Choukhande, Milind

N Dudhane. "Raktaja krimis (dermatophytes)" in Scientific Basis for Ayurvedic Therapies. Edited by Lakshmi Chandra Mishra. CRC press, Boca Raton, FL, 2004.

7 A K Panja, A Patra, S Choudhury, Abhichal Chattopadhyaya. The concept of antimicrobial activity in Ayurveda and the effect of some indigenous drugs on gram-negative bacteria. International Journal of Ayurvedic and Herbal Medicine (2011) 1(1): 1-7.

8 R B Hosamani. Infectious diseases – an Ayurvedic perspective. Health Sciences (2012) 1(1):1-8.

9 Nishant Shukla. Ayurvedic approach to communicable disease – an overview. Journal of Community Medicine & Health Education (2012). doi: 10.4172/scientificreports.122

10 Parameswarappa S Byadgi. Management of krimiroga as depicted in Charaka Samhita, Harita Samhita, Bhela Samhita and Bhaisajyaratnavali with current scientific outlook. Journal of Ayush: Ayurveda, Yoga, Unani, Siddha and Homeopathy (2013) 2(2): 25-31.

11 Rajesh Dabur, Amit Gupta, T K Mandal, Desh Deepak Singh, Vivek Bajpai, A M Gurav, G S Lavekar. Antimicrobial activity of some Indian medicinal plants. Afr. J. Trad. CAM (2007) 4(3): 313-318.

12 Mangesh Khond, J D Bhosale, Tasleem Arif, T K Mandal, M M Padhi, Rajesh Dabur. Screening of some selected medicinal plants extracts for in-vitro antimicrobial activity. Middle-East Journal of Scientific Research (2009) 4(4): 271-278.

13 K Nishteswar. Antimicrobial herbal drugs. International Research Journal of Pharmacy (2011) 2(12): 1-3.

14 Ramappa Raghavendra, Gurumurthy D Mahadevan. In vitro antimicrobial activity of various plant latex against resistant human pathogens. International Journal of Pharmacy and Pharmaceutical Sciences (2011) 3(4): 70-72.

15 Parmar Namita, Rawat Mukesh. Medicinal plants used as antimicrobial agents: a review. International Research Journal of Pharmacy (2012) 3(1):31-40.

16 P K Chaudhuri, Rashmi Srivastava, Sunil Kumar, Sushil Kumar. Phytotoxic and antimicrobial constituents of Bacopa monnieri and Holmskioldia sanguinea. Phytotherapy Research (2004) 18: 114-117.

17 T Ghosh, T K Maity, A Bose, G K Dash, M Das. A study on antimicrobial activity of Bacopa monnieri Linn. aerial parts. Journal of Natural Remedies (2006) 6(2): 170-173.

18 T Ghosh, T K Maity, A Bose, G K Dash, M Das. Antimicrobial activity of various fractions of ethanol extract of Bacopa monnieri Linn. aerial parts. Indian Journal of Pharmaceutical Sciences (2007) 69(2): 312-314.

19 Shyamapada Mandal, Manisha Deb Mandal, Nishith Kumar Pal. Antibacterial potential of Azadirachta indica seed and Bacopa monniera leaf extracts against multidrug resistant Salmonella enterica serovar typhi isolates. Arch Med Sci (2007) 3(1): 14-18.

20 P Sampathkumar, B Dheeba, V Vidhyasagar, T Arulprakash, R Vinothkannan. Potential antimicrobial activity of various extracts of Bacopa monnieri (Linn.). International Journal of Pharmacology (2008) 4(3): 230-

232.
21 S Sengupta, S N Ghosh, A K Das. Antimycotic potentiality of the plant extract of Bacopa monnieri (L.) Penn. Research Journal of Botany (2008) 3(2): 83-89.
22 Sharath Rajashekharappa, V Krishna, B N Sathyanarayana, Harish B Gowdar. Antibacterial activity of Bacoside-A – an active constituent isolated of Bacopa monnieri (L.) wettest. Pharmacologyonline (2008) 2: 517-528.
23 Abdul Viqar Khan, Qamar Uddin Ahmed, Indu Shukla, Athar Ali Khan. Antibacterial efficacy of Bacopa monnieri leaf extracts against pathogenic bacteria. Asian Biomedicine (2010) 4(4): 651-655.
24 S R Ayyappan, R Srikumar, R Thangaraj. Ophytochemical and antibacterial activity of Bacopa monniera against the common bacterial isolates from human. International Journal of Microbiological Research (2010) 1(2): 67-71.
25 Abhishek Mathur, Satish K Verma, Reena Purohit, Santosh K Singh, Deepika Mathur, G B K S Prasad, V K Dua. Pharmacological investigation of Bacopa monnieri on the basis of antioxidant, antimicrobial and anti-inflammatory properties. Journal of Chemical and Pharmaceutical Research (2010) 2(6): 191-198.
26 K Alam, N Parvez, S Yadav, K Molvi, N Hwisa, S M Al Sharif, D Pathak, Y Murthi, R Zafar. Antimicrobial activity of leaf callus of Bacopa monnieri L. Der Pharmacia Lettre (2011) 3(1): 287-291.
27 A K Azad, M Awang, M M Rahman. Phytochemical and microbiological evaluation of a local medicinal plant Bacopa monnieri (L.) Penn. International Journal of Current Pharmaceutical Review and Research (2012) 3(3): 66-78.
28 T Kalaivani, M Sasirekha, D Arunraj, V Palanichamy, C Rajasekaran. In vitro evaluation of antibacterial activity of phytochemical extracts from aerial parts of Bacopa monnieri (L) wettest (scorphulariaceae). Journal of Pharmacy Research (2012) 5(3): 1636-639.
29 S Vetriselvan, J Shankar, S Gayathiri, S Ishwin, C Hemah Devi, A Yaashini, G Sheerenjet. Comparative evaluation of in vitro antibacterial and antioxidant activity using standard drug and polyherbal formulation. International Journal of Phytopharmacology (2012) 3(2): 112-116.
30 Meghna Udgire, G R Pathade. Preliminary phytochemical and antifungal screening of crude extracts of the Bacopa monnieri. Universal Journal of Environmental Research and Technology (2012) 2(4): 347-354.

20 – Other Effects

In addition to the therapeutic effects described in the previous chapters, Brahmi has a number of other beneficial effects. Some of these are described in the following sections.

20.1 – Antinociceptive Activity

Shukia and coworkers[1] tested the antinociceptive activity of Brahmi rasayana (a polyherbal formulation of Bacopa monniera) in rats employing the hot wire method. Albino rats were treated with Brahmi rasayana (3, 10 or 30 g/kg, PO) and reaction times were recorded before the treatment and 30, 60, 120 and 180 min after the treatment. Brahmi rasayana at 3 and 10 g/kg showed antinociceptive effects at 120 and 180 min. At 30 g/kg, the effect was seen after all intervals.

Subhan and coworkers[2] examined the antinociceptive activity of a hydroethanolic extract (HE-ext) of Bacopa monniera in mice. The acetic acid-induced abdominal constriction assay and hot plate tests were conducted. Morphine and diclofenac were also examined for comparison. In the acetic acid-induced abdominal constriction assay, morphine, diclofenac and HE-ext showed a dose-dependent effect (morphine > diclofenac > HE-ext). Naloxone antagonized the effects of morphine and HE-ext. In the hot plate test, morphine produced an antinociceptive effect at all doses, HE-ext was effective only at 80 mg/kg, and diclofenac showed no effect. The antinociceptive effect of both morphine and HE-ext was antagonized by naloxone. The authors stated that "**the fact that BM HE-ext antinociception was naloxone reversible in both of these modalities also suggest that this action was opioid in nature.**"

Abbas and coworkers[3] showed the antinociceptive effect of an n-butanol extract of Bacopa monniera in mice employing the acetic acid induced writhing and hot plate tests. The antinociceptive effect was antagonized by naloxone in both tests, indicating an opioidergic mechanism. Another investigation[4] showed that oral administration of a hydroethanolic extract of Bacopa monniera to mice produced an antinociceptive effect in the acetic acid-induced writhing test that was not reversed by naloxone. Oral administration of HE-ext decreased locomotor activity, indicating a sedative effect, which was not antagonized by naloxone. The authors suggested that the antinociceptive and antilocomotive effects may be mediated through a non-opioidergic mechanism.

Biswas and coworkers[5] demonstrated the antinociceptive activity of an ethanol extract of Bacopa monniera (250 or 500 mg/kg) using the acetic acid induced writhing test in mice. The effect at 500 mg/kg was comparable to diclofenac at 25 mg/kg. Similar observations were made by Afjalus and coworkers[6].

Manju and Bhaskar[7] examined possible mechanisms of the antinociceptive activity of an aqueous extract of Bacopa monniera. The antinociceptive activity of AEBM was investigated in the presence and absence of yohimbine (a selective $\alpha 2$ receptor blocker), atenolol (a selective $\beta 1$ receptor blocker), cyproheptadine (a serotonin receptor antagonist) or naloxone (a non-selective opioid receptor antagonist) using various tests: acetic acid writhing tests with Swiss albino mice, formalin tests with Wistar rats and tail immersion tests with Swiss albino mice. The results are summarized below:

- In the acetic acid writhing test, AEBM (120 or 160 mg/kg, PO) showed antinociceptive activity, whereas neither yohimbine (1 mg/kg, i.p.) nor atenolol (1 mg/kg, i.p.) showed a significant effect. Both yohimbine and atenolol inhibited the effect of AEBM.
- In the formalin test, AEBM (80, 120 or 160 mg/kg, PO) showed antinociceptive activity, whereas cyproheptadine (1 mg/kg, i.p.) showed no significant effect. Cyproheptadine inhibited the effect of AEBM.
- In the tail immersion test, AEBM (160 mg/kg, PO) showed antinociceptive activity, whereas naloxone (2 mg/kg, i.p.) showed no significant effect. Naloxone inhibited the effect of AEBM.

The investigators concluded that endogenous adrenergic, serotonergic and opioidergic systems are involved in the analgesic mechanism of Bacopa monniera.

Vidya and coworkers[8] showed the antinociceptive activity of a polyherbal formulation (PHF) containing Bacopa monniera in rats using the tail immersion and hot plate tests.

Rauf and coworkers[9] investigated the effect of Bacopa monniera on the acquisition and expression of morphine tolerance in Balb C mice. An n-butanol fraction (n-Bt-ext) obtained from a methanol extract of Bacopa monniera was studied. The hot plate test was used to evaluate nociception. No tolerance to n-Bt-ext was observed in seven days of treatment. This study also revealed that the administration of n-Bt-ext along with morphine reduced both the expression and development of tolerance to morphine analgesia in mice.

Sumathi and coworkers[10] showed that an alcoholic extract of Bacopa monniera reduced in vitro effects of morphine withdrawal in the guinea-pig ileum.

20.2 – Mitigation of Harmful Effects of Cigarette Smoke

In a number of investigations, Anbarasi and coworkers[11-16] showed that bacoside A (BA) protected rats from harmful effects induced by exposure to cigarette smoke using the following experimental design. Adult male Wistar albino rats were divided into four groups and treated for 12 weeks as follows:

Group	Treatment
1	Control
2	Exposed to cigarette smoke for three hours, twice daily
3	BA (10 mg/kg/day, PO)
4	BA (10 mg/kg/day, PO), while exposed to cigarette smoke for three hours, twice daily

The animals were sacrificed and a number of biochemical analyses were done. Major observations from these investigations are summarized below:

- Group 2 showed increased LPO and cholesterol, and decreased phospholipid levels and mitochondrial enzymes in the brain compared to group 1. Group 4 showed a reversal of these changes[11].
- Group 2 showed increased LPO, sodium and calcium ions in the brain, and decreased activities of membrane bound ATPases and potassium and magnesium ions in the brain compared to group 1. Group 4 showed a reversal of these changes[12].
- CK and its isoforms (CK-MM, CK-MB, CK-BB)[13]:
  - Serum: Group 2 showed an increase compared to group 1. Group 4 showed a decrease compared to group 2.
  - Heart and brain: Group 2 showed a decrease compared to group 1. Group 4 showed an increase compared to group 2. CK and its isoforms have been used as sensitive markers of cardiac and cerebral damage.

- Group 2 showed decreased levels of both enzymatic and non-enzymatic antioxidants in the brain compared to group 1. Group 4 showed a reversal of these changes[14].
- Group 2 showed increased heat shock protein 70 kDa (Hsp 70) expression as well as induction of apoptosis in the brain compared to group 1. Group 4 showed a reversal of these changes. Induction of Hsp 70 by oxidants has been used as a marker for cell tissue injury.

  The investigators suggested that "**bacoside A likely provides potential means for developing effective preventive and/or therapeutic strategies in active and passive smokers.**"[15]
- Group 2 showed increased serum lactate dehydrogenase and its isoenzymes with a concomitant decrease of these in the lungs, heart, brain, liver and kidney compared to group 1. Group 4 did not show these changes[16].
- For each of these observations, there were no significant differences between groups 3 and 1.

20.3 – Prevention of DNA Damage

A number of investigations have shown the DNA protective effect of Bacopa monniera. Russo and coworkers[17] showed that a methanol extract of Bacopa monniera (BM) protected DNA from damage induced by H_2O_2 + UV-photolysis. DNA protection in human non-immortalized fibroblast cells was also studied.

A solution containing pBR322-derived DNA was subjected to H_2O_2 + UV-photolysis in the presence and absence of BM (800 μg/mL). In the absence of BM, the sample showed cleavage of scDNA to ocDNA and linDNA. Treatment with BM showed suppression of linDNA and partial recovery of scDNA. Experiments with the reference compounds trolox (200 μM) and ascorbic acid (200 μM) showed only suppression of linDNA.

Human non-immortalized fibroblast cells were treated with H_2O_2 in the presence and absence of BM (12 and 25 μg/mL). In the absence of BM, DNA showed damage and treatment with BM reduced the damage.

Garg and coworkers[18] found that a Bacopa monniera extract prevented γ-ray induced DNA damage. Bacopa monniera powder was extracted successively with methanol (BM), water-methanol (BAM) and water (BA). Solutions containing pBR322-derived DNA were irradiated in a ^{60}Co chamber with or without the extracts. Solutions of DNA without the extracts showed DNA damage and treatment with the extracts protected DNA in a dose-dependent manner. BAM was more effective than the other extracts.

Dhanasekaran and coworkers[19] showed that incubation of plasmid DNA in the presence of an alcoholic extract of Bacopa monniera (0-10 μg) for one hour showed no effect on the supercoiled conformation of DNA.

Anand and coworkers[20] showed that methanol and water extracts of Bacopa monniera protected DNA (derived from the pRSETA plasmid) from H_2O_2 + UV induced damage. The methanol extract was found to be more effective than the water extract.

20.4 – Broncho-Vasodilatory and Mast Cell Stabilizing Activities

In vitro and animal studies have demonstrated the broncho-vasodilatory and mast cell stabilizing effects of Bacopa monniera. These studies validate the use of Brahmi in Ayurveda to treat asthma, bronchitis, and a number of other respiratory diseases.

Dar and Channa[21] showed that an ethanol extract of Bacopa monniera (100-700 μg/mL) induced a relaxant effect on the ring segments of pulmonary arteries (guinea pigs and rabbits), aorta (rabbits) and trachea preparations (guinea pigs) in a dose-dependent manner. Pretreatment of the blood vessels (rabbits and guinea pigs) with atropine did not change the relaxant effect induced by BM, indicating the absence of muscarinic receptor activation. Pretreatment of the blood vessels with propranolol did not change the relaxant effect induced by BM, indicating that β-adrenoceptors were not stimulated. Pretreatment of the tracheal preparation with propranolol partially blocked the relaxant effect induced by BM, indicating activation of β2-adrenoceptors. The relaxant effect induced by BM in all tissues was inhibited by pretreatment with indomethacin, indicating involvement of the cyclooxygenase pathway. In a subsequent investigation, Channa and Dar[22] showed that an ethanol extract of Bacopa monniera antagonized the bronchoconstrictor action of carbachol in anesthetized rats.

Channa and coworkers[23] examined the bronchovasodilatory activity of an ethanol extract of Bacopa monniera and its various fractions, sub-fractions, sub-sub fractions and a pure constituent (betulinic acid). The results are summarized below:

- The PE, CH_2Cl_2, methanol and aqueous fractions inhibited carbachol-induced bronchoconstriction, hypotension and bradycardia in anesthetized rats. The methanol fraction was more effective in inhibiting both tracheal pressure and blood pressure compared to the other fractions.

- The $CHCl_3$/methanol sub-fraction showed a greater inhibitory effect on tracheal pressure and blood pressure compared to other sub-fractions.
- The sub-sub fraction as well as betulinic acid inhibited carbachol-induced changes on tracheal pressure, blood pressure and heart rate. Betulinic acid (0.228 mg/kg) was more effective than the sub-sub fraction (2.5 mg/kg).

Mast cells play an important role in allergic reactions, and mast cell stabilizers are indicated in the management of various allergic disorders. Samiulla and coworkers[29] evaluated the mast cell stabilizing activity of various extracts of Bacopa monniera (petroleum ether, chloroform, methanol and water). Disodium cromoglycate (a well-known mast cell stabilizer) was used as a reference standard. All of the extracts showed mast cell stabilizing activity. The methanol extract was the most powerful and its effect was comparable to disodium cromoglycate.

20.5 – Spasmolytic Activity

Bacopa monniera has demonstrated spasmolytic activity and is beneficial in the management of irritable bowel syndrome (IBS).

Dar and Channa[24] found that an ethanol extract of Bacopa monniera inhibited the spontaneous movements of the guinea pig ileum and rabbit jejunum. The extract inhibited acetylcholine- and histamine-induced contraction in the guinea pig ileum, indicating direct action of the extract on smooth muscles. The extract attenuated responses induced by $CaCl_2$ in the blood vessels and jejunum of rabbits. The extract had no effect on noradrenaline- or caffeine-induced contraction. The investigators stated that "**spasmolytic effect of the B. monniera extract in smooth muscles is predominantly due to inhibition of calcium influx via both voltage and receptor operated calcium channels of the cell membrane.**"

Recently, Channa and Dar[25] demonstrated the calcium channel blocking activity of an ethanol extract of Bacopa monniera in guinea pig tracheal smooth muscles. The extract suppressed calcium-induced responses non-competitively like nifedipine, a known calcium channel blocker.

Yadav and coworkers[26] evaluated the therapeutic efficacy of an Ayurvedic preparation containing Aegle marmelos Correa and Bacopa monniera in the management of IBS. In a double-blind, randomized, placebo-controlled trial, 169 patients were treated with the Ayurvedic preparation, a standard drug, or placebo for 6 weeks. The Ayurvedic formulation was effective in 65% of its cases, the standard drug was 78% effective, and the placebo was 33% effective. The ayurvedic formulation was more effective in patients with diarrhea. Relapse rates at 6 months were similar in all groups.

20.6 – Antihypothyroid Activity

Kar and coworkers[27] showed that an extract of Bacopa monniera (50% ethanol) augmented thyroid hormone concentration in mice. Swiss albino male mice treated with the extract by gastric intubation for 15 days (200 mg/kg/day) showed increased serum concentration of the thyroid hormone T4 (41%) compared to the control group. No significant change in T3 was observed. The investigators suggested that the extract might directly stimulate synthesis and/or release of T4 at the glandular level.

20.7 – Antifertility Activity

Singh and Singh[28] showed that an aqueous extract of Bacopa monniera caused reversible suppression of spermatogenesis and fertility in mice without producing systemic toxicity.

References

1 Bina Shukia, N K Khanna, J L Godhwani. Effect of Brahmi rasayan on the central nervous system. Journal of Ethnopharmacology (1987) 21: 65-74.

2 F Subhan, M Abbas, K Rauf, M Arfan, R D E Sewell, G Ali. The role of opioidergic mechanisms in the activity of Bacopa monnieri extract against tonic and acute phasic pain modalities. Pharmacologyonline (2010) 3: 903-914.

3 M Abbas, F Subhan, N Mohani, K Rauf, G Ali, M Khan. The involvement of opioidergic mechanisms in the activity of Bacopa monnieri extract and its toxicological studies. Afr. J Pharm. Pharmacol. (2011) 5(8): 1120-1124.

4 Muzaffar Abbas, Fazal Subhan, Khalid Rauf, Ikram-Ul-Haq, Syed Nadeem-UL-Hassan Mohani. The involvement of non opioidergic mechanism in the antinociceptive and antilocomotive activity of Bacopa monnieri. Iranian Journal of Pharmacology and Therapeutics (2012) 11(1): 15-19.

5 S K Biswas, J Das, A Chowdhury, U K Karmakar, H Hossain. Evaluation of antinociceptive and antioxidant activities of whole plant extract of Bacopa monniera. Res. J Med. Plant (2012) 6(8): 607-614.

6 S Md. Afjalus, N Chakma, M Rahman, M Salahuddin, S S Kumar. Assessment of analgesic, antidiarrhoeal and cytotoxic activity of ethanolic extract of the whole plant of Bacopa monnieri Linn. IRJP (2012) 3(10): 98-101.

7 Manju Bhaskar, A G Jagtap. Exploring the possible mechanisms of action

behind the antinociceptive activity of Bacopa monniera. International Journal of Ayurveda Research (2011) 2(1): 2-7.

8 S Vidya, D Sravya, P Neeraja, A Ramesh. Evaluation of anti-inflammatory and analgesic activity of poly herbal formulation (PHF) in albino rats. International Journal of Research in Pharmaceutical Sciences (2011) 2(3): 444-449.

9 Khalid Rauf, Fazal Subhan, Muzaffar Abbas, Amir Badshah, Ihsan Ullah, Sami Ullah. Effect of bacosides on acquisition and expression of morphine tolerance. Phytomedicine (2011) 18: 836-842.

10 T Sumathi, M Nayeem, K Balakrishna, G Veluchamy, S N Devaraj. Alcoholic extract of Bacopa monniera reduces the in vitro effects of morphine withdrawal in guinea-pig ileum. Journal of Ethnopharmacology (2002) 82(2-3) 75-81.

11 K Anbarasi, G Vani, C S Devi. Protective effect of bacoside A on cigarette smoking-induced brain mitochondrial dysfunction in rats. J. Environ Pathol Toxicol Oncol (2005) 24(3): 225-234.

12 K Anbarasi, G Vani, K Balakrishna, C S Shyamala Devi. Effect of bacoside A on membrane-bound ATPases in the brain of rats exposed to cigarette smoke. J. Biochem Molecular Toxicology (2005) 19(1): 59-65.

13 K Anbarasi, G Vani, K Balakrishna, C S Shyamala Devi. Creatine kinase isoenzyme patterns upon chronic exposure to cigarette smoke: protective effect of bacoside A. Vascular Pharmacology (2005) 42: 57-61.

14 K Anbarasi, G Vani, K Balakrishna, C S Shyamala Devi. Effect of bacoside A on brain antioxidant status in cigarette smoke exposed rats. Life Sciences (2006) 78: 1378-1384.

15 K Anbarasi, G Kathirvel, G Vani, G Jayaraman, C S Shyamala Devi. Cigarette smoking induces heat shock protein 70 kDa expression and apotosis in rat brain: modulation by bacoside A. Neuroscience (2006) 138: 1127-1135.

16 Kothandapani Anbarasi, Kuruvimalai Ekambaram Sabitha, Chennam Srinivasulu Shyamala Devi. Lactate dehydrogenase isoenzyme patterns upon chronic exposure to cigarette smoke: protective effect of bacoside A. Environmental Toxicology and Pharmacology. (2005) 20(2): 345-350.

17 Alessandra Russo, Angelo A Izzo, Francesca Borrelli, Marcella Renis, Angelo Vanella. Free radical scavenging capacity and protective effect of Bacopa monniera L. on DNA damage. Phytotherapy Research (2003) 17: 870-875.

18 A N Garg, A Kumar, A G C Nair, A V R Reddy. Elemental analysis of Brahmi (Bacopa monnieri) extracts by neutron activation and its bioassay for antioxidant, radio protective and anti-lipid peroxidation activity. J Radional Nucl Chem (2009) 281: 53-58.

19 Muralikrishnan Dhanasekaran, Binu Tharakan, Leigh A Holcomb, Angie R Hitt, Keith A Young, Bala V Manyam. Neuroprotective mechanisms of Ayurvedic antidementia botanical Bacopa monniera. Phytotherapy Research (2007) 21: 965-969.

20 Anand T, Mahadeva Naika, Swamy M S L, Farhath Khanum. Antioxidant and DNA damage preventive properties of Bacopa monniera (L) wettst. Free Radicals and Antioxidants (2011) 1(1): 84-90.

---

21 Ahsana Dar, Shabana Channa. Relaxant effect of ethanol extract of Bacopa monniera on trachea, pulmonary artery and aorta from rabbit and guinea-pig. Phytotherapy research (1997) 2:323-325.

22 A Dar, S Channa. Bronchodilatory and cardiovascular effects of an ethanol extract of Bacopa monniera in anaesthetized rats. Phytomedicine (1997) 4(4): 319-323.

23 Shabana Channa, Ahsana Dar, Muhammad Yaqoob, Shazia Anjum, Zia Sultani, Atta-ur-Rahman. Broncho-vasodilatory activity of fractions and pure constituents isolated from Bacopa monniera. Journal of Ethnopharmacology (2003) 86: 27-35.

24 Ahsana Dar, Shabana Channa. Calcium antagonistic activity of Bacopa monniera on vascular and intestinal smooth muscles of rabbit guinea-pig. Journal of Ethnopharmacology (1999) 66: 167-174.

25 Shabana Channa, Ahsana Dar. Calcium antagonistic activity of Bacopa monniera in guinea-pig trachea. Indian Journal of pharmacology (2012) 44(4): 516-518.

26 S K Yadav, A K Jain, S N Tripathi, J P Gupta. Irritable bowel syndrome: therapeutic evaluation of indigenous drugs. The Indian journal of medical research (1989) 90: 496-503.

27 A Kar, S Panda, S Bharti. Relative efficacy of three medicinal plant extracts in the alteration of thyroid hormone concentrations in male mice. Journal of Ethnopharmacology (2002) 81: 281-285.

28 Akanksha Singh, Shio Kumar Singh. Evaluation of antifertility potential of Brahmi in male mouse. Contraception (2009) 79: 71-79.

29 D S Samiulla, D Prashanth, A Amit. Mast cell stabilising activity of Bacopa monnieri. Fitoterapia (2001) 72: 284-285.

21 – Safety-Related Issues and Conclusion

21.1 – General

Brahmi has had centuries of clinical usage in Ayurvedic medicine. It has an excellent safety profile, being well-tolerated at pharmacological doses and not exhibiting serious adverse side effects. A number of animal and clinical trials have been recently conducted to evaluate the toxicity, safety and side effects of Bacopa monniera.

21.2 – Toxicity Studies

Martis and coworkers[1] conducted acute toxicity studies in male albino Wistar rats of aqueous and alcoholic extracts of Bacopa monniera administered both orally and intraperitoneally. LD_{50} values for i.p. administration were 1 and 15 g/kg for the aqueous and alcoholic extracts, respectively. For oral administration, the alcoholic extract had an LD_{50} of 17 g/kg, and the aqueous extract did not show any toxicity up to a dose of 5 g/kg.

Giri and Khan[2] evaluated bacosides A and B for genotoxic activities in Swiss albino mice. Mice treated with bacosides A and B (20, 40 or 80 mg/kg, i.p.) did not show significant differences in chromosomal aberration, sister chromatid exchange and micronuclei formation compared to the corresponding control group. The LD_{50} value was 300 mg/kg.

Allan and coworkers[3] evaluated the toxicity of BacoMind in Sprague Dawley rats. The LD_{50} of a single oral administration was found to be 2400 mg/kg. In a 14 day repeated dose study, oral treatment with BacoMind was well-tolerated without observable adverse side effects up to the dose of 500 mg/kg. Also, administration of BacoMind (85-500 mg/kg, PO) for 90 days did not show any evidence of toxicity.

Vidya and coworkers[4] investigated the acute toxicity of a polyherbal formulation (PHF) containing Bacopa monniera leaves, Aegle marmelos leaves and Eugenia jambolana seeds. Albino rats were treated with the PHF (50-2000 mg/kg, i.p.). No mortality was observed after 24 hours, but after 48 hours, mortality was observed at 1000 and 2000 mg/kg.

Ghosh and coworkers[5] treated Swiss albino mice with an ethanol extract of Bacopa monniera (100-3000 mg/kg, PO) and observed the animals for 14 days. No mortality occurred during this period.

21.3 – Safety (Clinical Trials)

Singh and Dhawan[6] evaluated the safety of pharmacological doses of bacoside A and B in healthy male adults through a double blind, placebo-controlled phase I clinical trial. Administration of a single dose of bacoside A and B (20 to 300 mg, PO) was well tolerated with no observable adverse side effects. Clinical, hematological and biochemical examination of patients before and after the trial showed no significant differences.

Pravina and coworkers[7] conducted a 30-day phase I clinical trial for the safety evaluation of BacoMind. Healthy adults were given a 300 mg dose of BacoMind once a day for the first 15 days, and a 450 mg dose once a day for the next 15 days. Clinical, hematological, biochemical and electrocardiographic examination before and after the trial showed no significant differences. No major adverse effects were reported during the trial.

Bacopa monniera is not recommended for pregnant and breastfeeding women, since no safety studies are available.

21.4 – Side Effects

Bacopa monniera is generally considered safe at pharmacological doses. However, a number of mild side effects listed below have been reported[8-10]:

- Dry mouth
- Excessive thirst
- Nausea
- Palpitations
- Gastrointestinal tract cramps
- Indigestion
- Increased stool frequency
- Flu-like symptoms

21.5 – Herb-Drug Interactions

Concerns have emerged recently around herb-drug interactions, especially in older adults who commonly use herbal supplements along with prescription and/or nonprescription drugs. Herb-drug interactions have both a pharmacokinetic (absorption, distribution and excretion of a drug) and pharmacodynamic (pharmacological activities) basis. These interactions may occur through inhibition of hepatic and intestinal drug-metabolizing enzymes (e.g. cytochrome P450) and drug transporters (e.g. p-glycoprotein)[14].

Interactions of several popular herbs with commonly used prescription drugs have been reported[11-13], but Bacopa monniera's interactions with conventional drugs has not been studied extensively. The limited amount of information available is presented below. Bacopa monniera has been observed to:

- **Have anxiolytic and antidepressant activity, as described in Chapter 8**
- **Have anticonvulsant activity, as described in Chapter 10**
- **Inhibit cytochrome P enzymes[14,15].** BM preparations should be used cautiously with drugs that are cleared via CYP2C19, CYP2C9, CYPIA2 and CYP3A4 catalyzed metabolism.
- **Block calcium channels, as described in Chapter 20**
- **Augment thyroid hormone synthesis, as described in Chapter 20**
- **Cause reversible suppression of spermatogenesis and fertility, as described in Chapter 20**

In all of these cases, dosage should be carefully monitored when Bacopa monniera is used as an adjuvant treatment.

21.6 – Concluding Remarks

Overall, the results obtained from numerous experiments strongly indicate the beneficial effects of Brahmi in the treatment/management of various disorders/diseases as observed in Ayurveda. In particular, Brahmi shows great promise as a safe and efficacious nootropic in both normal and dementia models. However, results obtained by different investigators using similar extracts and identical experimental designs diverge significantly, leading to some confusion in interpretation. This is not unexpected, as there are a number of variables to control that can influence the composition of the herb. These variables include the environment and soil in which the plant was grown, season of harvest, age of the plant, as well as on how the harvested material was processed. It is important to characterize the material used in studies as thoroughly as possible. In view of the positive results observed so far, it is worthwhile to continue both basic research and clinical trials. Trials with longer durations should be conducted to establish the safety and efficacy of Brahmi.

References

1 Gladys Martis A Rao, K S Karanth. Neuropharmacological activity of Herpestis monniera. Fitoterapia (1992) 63(5): 399-404.

2 Ashok Kumar Giri, Kaleem Ahmed Khan. Chromosome aberrations, sister chromatid exchange and micronuclei formation analysis in mice after in vivo exposure to bacoside A and B. Cytologia (1996) 61: 99-103.

3 Allan J Joshua, A Damodaran, N S Deshmukh, K S Goudar, A Amit. Safety evaluation of standardized phytochemical composition extracted from Bacopa monnieri in Sprague-Dawley rats. Food and Chemical Toxicology (2007) 45(10): 1928-37.

4 S Vidya, D Sravya, P Neeraja, A Ramesh. Evaluation of anti-inflammatory and analgesic activity of poly herbal formulation (PHF) in albino rats. International Journal of Research in Pharmaceutical Sciences (2011) 2(3): 444-449.

5 Tirtha Ghosh, Tapan Kumar Maity, Mrinmay Das, Anindya Bose, Deepak Kumar Dash. In vitro antioxidant and hepatoprotective activity of ethanolic extract of Bacopa monnieri Linn. aerial parts. IJPT (2007) 6(1): 77-85.

6 H K Singh, B N Dhawan. Neuropsychopharmacological effects of the Ayurvedic nootropic Bacopa monniera Linn (Brahmi). Indian Journal of Pharmacology (1997) 29(5): 359-365.

7 K Pravina, K R Ravindra, K S Goudar, D R Vinod, A J Joshua, P Wasim, K Venkateshwarlu, V S Saxena, A Amit. Safety evaluation of BacoMind in healthy volunteers: a phase I study. Phytomedicine (2007) 14: 301-308.

8 C Stough, J Loyd, J Clarke, L A Downey, C W Hutchison, T Rodgers, P J Nathan. The chronic effects of an extract of Bacopa monniera (Brahmi) on cognitive function in healthy human subjects. Psychopharmacology (2001) 156: 481-484.

9 Carlo Calabrese, William L Gregory, Michael Leo, Dale Kraemer, Kerry Bone, Barry Oken. Effects of a standardized Bacopa monnieri extract on cognitive performance, anxiety and depression in the elderly: a randomized double-blind, placebo-controlled trial. The Journal of Alternative and Complementary Medicine (2008) 14(6): 707-713.

10 Annette Morgan, John Stevens. Does Bacopa monnieri improve memory performance in older persons? Results of a randomized, placebo-controlled double-blind trial. The Journal of Alternative and Complementary Medicine (2010) 16(7): 753-759.

11 Bill J Gurley, Dorothy W Hagan. "Herbal and dietary supplement interactions with drugs." in Handbook of Food-Drug Interactions. Edited by B J McCabe, E H Frankel, J J Wolfe, CRC Press, Boca Raton, 2003.

12 Y W Francis Lam, Shiew-Mei Huang, Stephen D Hall. Herbal Supplements-Drug Interactions: Scientific and Regulatory Perspectives. Taylor & Francis, 2006.

13 Amitava Dasgupta, and Catherine A. Hammett-Stabler. Herbal Supplements: Efficacy, Toxicity, Interactions with Western Drugs, and Effects on Clinical Laboratory Tests. John Wiley & Sons, 2011.

14 Seetha Ramasamy, Lik Voon Kiew, Lip Yong Chung. Inhibition of human Cytochrome P450 enzymes by Bacopa monnieri standardized extract and constituents. Molecules (2014) 19(2): 2588-2601.

15 Rajbir Singh, Jagadeesh Panduri, Devendra Kumar, Deepak Kumar, Hardik Chandsana, Rachumallu Ramakrishna, Rabi Sankar Bhatta. Evaluation of memory enhancing clinically available standardized extract of Bacopa monniera on P-glycoprotein and Cytochrome P450 3A in Sprague-Dawley rats. PLOS ONE (2013) 8(8): e72517.

Common Abbreviations

5-HT – serotonin
6-OHDA – 6-hydroxydopamine
ACh – acetylcholine
AChE – acetylcholinesterase
ALP – alkaline phosphatase
ALT – alanine aminotransferase
AST – aspartate aminotransferase
ATP – adenosine triphosphate
CAT – catalase
CK – creatine kinase
DA – dopamine
DMSO – dimethyl sulfoxide
EtOAc – ethyl acetate
GABA – gamma aminobutyric acid
GOT – glutamate oxaloacetate transaminase
GPT – glutamate pyruvate transaminase
GPx – glutathione peroxidase
GR – glutathione reductase
GSH – glutathione
GST – glutathione-S-transferase
HP – hydroperoxide
LDH – lactate dehydrogenase
LHP – lipid hydroperoxide
LPO – lipid peroxidation
MAO – monoamine oxidase
MDA – malondialdehyde
n-BuOH – n-butanol
NMDA – N-methyl-D-aspartate
PC – protein carbonyl
PND – postnatal day
ROS – reactive oxygen species
RNS – reactive nitrogen species
SOD – superoxide dismutase

www.ingramcontent.com/pod-product-compliance
Lightning Source LLC
Chambersburg PA
CBHW070409270326
41926CB00014B/2765

9780984381227